The MOTTO Effect

*Transforming Hashimoto's with
10 powerful health & lifestyle MOTTOs*

Copyright © 2020 by Meena Chan

All rights reserved. No part of this book may be reproduced or used in any manner without the prior written permission of the copyright owner. The only exception is brief quotations in printed reviews.

DEDICATION

To my parents, my in laws, my wonderful husband Aravind and my adorable children Kavin and Tara, who always believed in me and have helped me become who I am today.

To my dear Hashimoto-ers.

CONTENTS

Foreword 1

Introduction 5

Part I: Hello Moto

CHAPTER ONE
The Sugarcane Machine 12

CHAPTER TWO
The Revolving Door 16

CHAPTER THREE
The Dancing Samurai's 24

Part II: Stumbling Onto MOTTO

CHAPTER FOUR
Google Guided 38

CHAPTER FIVE
Expansive Awareness 44

CHAPTER SIX
Intentionally Me 55

CHAPTER SEVEN
Trip Over Transition 62

Part III: Discovering My MOTTO's

The Body MOTTO 70

> CHAPTER EIGHT
> The Moto MOTTO 72
>
> CHAPTER NINE
> The Yogic MOTTO 84
>
> CHAPTER TEN
> The Plateful MOTTO 100
>
> CHAPTER ELEVEN
> The Marma MOTTO 118

The Mind MOTTO 130

> CHAPTER TWELVE
> The Zen MOTTO 132
>
> CHAPTER THIRTEEN
> The Hola MOTTO 143
>
> CHAPTER FOURTEEN
> The Digital Sunset MOTTO 152
>
> CHAPTER FIFTEEN
> The Reasoning MOTTO 159

The Soul MOTTO 169

CHAPTER SIXTEEN
The Golden Hour 171

CHAPTER SEVENTEEN
The Supreme MOTTO 183

Author's Note 189

Acknowledgements 190

Notes 191

FOREWORD

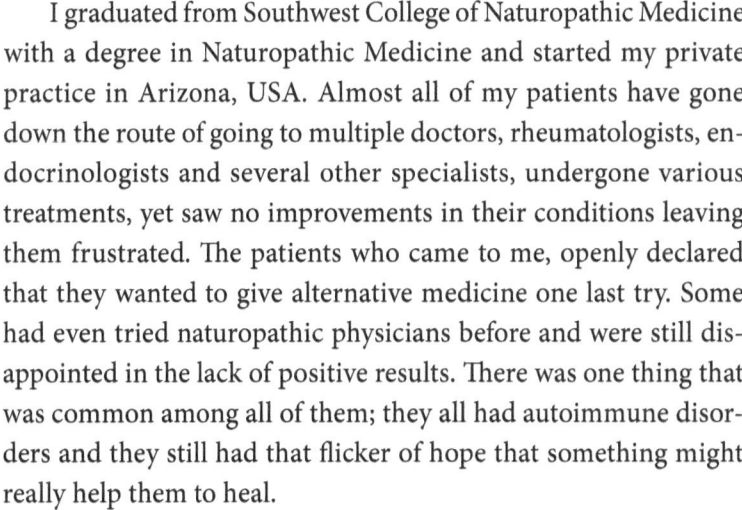

I graduated from Southwest College of Naturopathic Medicine with a degree in Naturopathic Medicine and started my private practice in Arizona, USA. Almost all of my patients have gone down the route of going to multiple doctors, rheumatologists, endocrinologists and several other specialists, undergone various treatments, yet saw no improvements in their conditions leaving them frustrated. The patients who came to me, openly declared that they wanted to give alternative medicine one last try. Some had even tried naturopathic physicians before and were still disappointed in the lack of positive results. There was one thing that was common among all of them; they all had autoimmune disorders and they still had that flicker of hope that something might really help them to heal.

Autoimmune conditions in general, affect a large population in the United States, and one of the most common ones is Hashimoto's thyroiditis. The current guideline to manage Hashimoto's thyroiditis treatment is to simply check the TSH levels in the blood, and if it is within the recommended range by conventional lab standard, the patients are considered 'normal'. However, they might not feel 'normal' in any way. Patients' diet, lifestyle and potential triggers for autoimmunity are never considered (despite all of the published research articles). When patients come to me, I can relate to them very well, as I had watched my mother go through excruciating rheumatoid arthritis when I was studying for medicine. She was put on three different harsh medications but continued to suffer with severe joint pains. My mother continued to live taking pain medications and it left me feeling like a helpless bystander. After completing years of education, in both alternative and conventional medicine, I was determined to find a solution for my mother. I read all of the books I could find written by holistic and functional healthcare providers (MDs, NDs, DCs), and slowly I realized that there were better solutions – there were alternative methods to improving a patient's quality of life with no invasive drugs or procedures. My mother's harrowing experience paved the way for my career; I discovered my passion for global wellness and community health.

My first advice to anyone suffering with an autoimmune disease is to do everything to take full control of your health. Your health is your responsibility and should not be in the hands of another medical provider. Physicians are there to help and guide you, but ultimately you know what works for your body. Be open-minded and seek out physicians who truly care about you - MD, DO, ND, or DC. Find providers that use an evidence-based integrative medical approach to address not only the symptoms of autoimmune attack, but those who also look at your lifestyle holistically, and treat the root cause. The immune system is complex and no one has all the answers, but with the right team behind you (including your family), you don't have to feel hopeless or disempowered.

There are providers who claim they can heal you with their "protocol" which would be the one stop solution for everyone. Are all autoimmune patients the same? The answer to this is a big NO. I can list hundreds of triggers and causes for autoimmunity; so how can a standard "protocol" address them all? If there is one, the person invented it should have already won the Nobel Prize in medicine. If you go to a provider who claims that all autoimmune conditions start with a "leaky gut", or that "leaky gut" must be addressed first before you recover; challenge them by asking for research based evidence. I know leaky gut has become the new trend in alternative and functional medicine, and I do admit that a lot of the times it does play a role in autoimmunity, but without thorough investigation, never jump into a standardized protocol, or focus only on the gut for complete recovery. 80% of a physician's job is to investigate, discover the mechanism of disease formation, learn all about the patient's lifestyle and triggers and explain that process thoroughly to patients with evidence. The other 20%, is to work with the patients and provide them an individualized solution. Thanks to all of the researchers who have worked tirelessly on developing functional medicine oriented laboratories, and treatment options, has meant that the recovery path has opened up greatly, so patients need not suffer in silence.

When I first met Meena, she had gone through a devastating health journey as well, and seemed to be in a lot of pain. She had shrunken in size, had sunken eyes, came to me with a long list of symptoms and her fatigue was so debilitating, that even visits to the physician demanded a lot from her. However, what I admired in her, was her willingness to learn and she always seemed hopeful that the right cure was coming her way. It was a learning experience for me as well as to how to educate patients and empower them. Today, she's bountiful, full of joy and energy, with a never fading smile and has a great sense of humor (she always did, even when she was downright sick!). I'm extremely proud of her to see her transformational journey, and how far she's come along in her healing and recovering. When we last checked her thyroid, her antibodies had reduced drastically and she is still in remission and no longer suffers ill health. Not only has she healed herself, she surprised me by writing this book. I can greatly recommend this read to anyone suffering from Hashimoto's, or from any other autoimmune condition, as they can highly benefit from this book. This is her personal testimonial and anyone reading this will be able to relate to it. Use this as your beginner's guide to learning more about this illness and ask questions, because if you don't, no-one will provide the answers. I read it with much interest as she navigates through the mind, body and soul and has provided a tremendous wealth of information in a simple and easy to understand manner. Ultimately, the illness needs to be looked at holistically, and to my knowledge, she is the first one to have broken it down so beautifully in the mind, body and soul parameters, and to provide an exact methodology within each of those categories to begin with. As a physician, reading from a patient's perspective as to what they underwent, was eye opening. For this reason, I really wish for more patients were to write about their personal journeys, otherwise it would all be medical jargons if it were to come from physicians! The book includes a good dose of inspiration, guidance, humor and is an emotionally touching read.

Have fun reading,

Dr. YiQiu Hu

Doctor of Naturopathic Medicine

Co-founder and Medical Director,
of a leading medical practice in Arizona, USA.

INTRODUCTION

Absolute stillness made me nervous.

I tried to walk across the room, then I laid down uncomfortably on my side, before I restlessly shifted myself onto my back. As I gulped down a glass of water, I felt the surge of anxiety growing within me. I was gripped in uneasiness by the stillness, and shining a flashlight on my tummy made no difference. There was still no movement and the deep concern I had begun to feel worsened. I played soothing music and even tried to talk to my baby, hoping that my voice would make him react but nothing created a response from him that day. I could not afford to be careless; I was on the home stretch, the 38th week of my pregnancy. As new parents, we knew no better and we rushed to the hospital. The doctors decided on using an electrocardiogram (ECG) and an ultrasound to monitor the baby. I felt queasy when the bigger machines were placed next to me, and as the nurse added the straps around my belly. As soon as the straps were on, my son moved. "The baby was fine!" The relief we felt in that moment was enormous and I felt tears well up in my eyes. After a few more rounds of tests, we were almost finished with the checkups.

The chief doctor walked into the examination room and explained to us that he had heard a mild heart murmur and due to the baby's position, a normal delivery may not be possible. The best alternative then was to have a caesarean delivery. His announcement caught me off guard and shook me up, I had not imagined a caesarean even in my strangest dream; my heart sank in despair and I felt a sense of disappointment. My train of thoughts was once again interrupted, but this time the doctor's voice had an urgency "this is an emergency cesarean, there's not much time left to think, we need to act fast." My husband and I signed the paperwork to proceed with the caesarean delivery as quickly as possible. The circumstances were most unsettling as we thought we would have been in and out of the hospital after a few checkups, but now we would be there for a few days. I felt overwhelmed and unprepared; all of a sudden, our new reality was sinking in. I was placed on a stretcher and was wheeled into the operating theatre. Moments later, I was transferred to the table with bright flashing lights above me. The doctors and nurses wore their clinical masks and gloves; my husband was by my side supporting me and tightly held my hands.

"1 scissors, 6 tissue forceps, 1 serrated forceps…"

The countdown began and the voices faded away - I was knocked out unconscious. It had been an excruciatingly long day.

I was woken up by my son's cry, this tiny being with a head full of hair, batting his beautiful long eye lashes as we locked eyes with each other briefly for the first time. He looked as shocked as I felt. The sight of my baby and the tremendous relief at knowing that he was safe and healthy created a few minutes of feeling euphoric, overriding the lasting effects of the sedation I had received not so long before. At that moment nothing else mattered, as I had the little world in my hands, my son was born!

THE BIRTH OF THE MOTTO EFFECT

My son's birth marked the beginning of postpartum thyroiditis (PPT). After my second child, the condition became full-blown, rocking the very foundation of my life. The journey began with me being diagnosed with Hashimoto's thyroiditis; an autoimmune disorder. The illness progressed rapidly leaving me with a multitude of debilitating symptoms, and a frantic search to recover. As a new parent, with a full-time job, managing my family and household, having the time and energy to work on my symptoms and recovery was not easy. I could not understand the medical terminologies and each visit to the doctor meant that I had to do a lot of research, homework and prepare a list of questions to ask - only to return from the doctor's visit with many more questions than I would have had earlier. I was too brain fogged to search through the internet or even to look up and read parts of gigantic books. It left me deeply frustrated with the whole process and I longed for a quick recovery. I did everything that was in my favor and was diligent with my medications and doctor appointments, yet I felt I was letting life pass by me with no real recovery in sight. My body was failing, but I had to take care of two little kids who were dependent on me, so the urgency of my situation left me desperate to heal.

> *Even though Autoimmune disorders are growing at an alarming rate, with more than 1 in 12 suffering from an Autoimmune disorder and it is one of the most common categories of illness ahead of cancer or heart disease. They are 3 times more common now than they were decades ago with over 75% being affected women.*

However, I did not know whom to approach for help or what my next steps were. I hoped for an answer - if only there was a one stop guide to look into, that would be the be-all-and-end-all, as well as the cure for all of this madness I was going through.

Taking one baby step at a time, I slowly discovered what was working for my body, expanded my awareness to my mind and then reached the pristine place – my soul. I strongly believe if something has come into your life, then there is a bigger purpose. Little did I know that when I was first diagnosed with Hashimoto's, my life would change so much for the better. The autoimmune disorder brought about greater order into my life, that might have not been otherwise. I would have continued with raising my kids and working a full-time job, not really giving life much deeper thought or meaning. My life transformed in all aspects and I developed a tremendous sense of gratitude, the more I thought about what an amazing blessing in disguise this journey had been.

The MOTTO Effect is here to give you hope and the belief that a recovery is possible from autoimmune disorders. Many western practitioners believe that a recovery is absolutely not possible and that the only way is to take the medications. I do agree partly, that medications are needed to control the thyroid imbalances; however, medications alone will not be the one-step solution to complete recovery.

> *The journey to wellness starts first with a single step of believing you can overcome.*

The MOTTO Effect is all about choosing your mindset or your perspective. Nature's most powerful lesson on transformation comes in the form of a butterfly; the transformation of the caterpillar to the butterfly teaches us not to quit before the beautiful journey begins. You could stay stuck in Hashimoto's, or if you want to redefine Hashimoto's, develop your own life transforming MOTTOs - to overcome, become and recover from the autoimmune illness similar to the caterpillar. **From a moto to MOTTO, you are only short of the letter 'T', which is the transformation.** Simple lifestyle changes can alter the way you live, which in turn will impact you and your family, and will lead to overall wellbeing. Think of this as a mental switch and each time it's off, the Hashimoto's kicks in - you'll feel like laying down and sleeping forever - when you switch on the MOTTO Effect, you'll want to do what's needed, irrespective of how your body feels.

Combining a good dose of ancient eastern practices in the

modern western world that we live in, The MOTTO Effect will help you navigate through this most difficult period by helping you make the conscious right choices. You too, may also have the added stress of being a new parent to take into account or life changing events or other stressful situations that life does throw up. Not a single person should be left helpless and hopeless, frustrated and desperate and not knowing what to do or whom to reach out to. This book is designed to help guide you through your journey and offer the much needed inspiration and support that you may greatly need in these times. It's my sincere hope that the MOTTO method that I created helps you in bringing back order into your life, just like it did for me, and for this to be the magical guide to all my Hashimoto-ers; the guide that I once longed would be available for me. When I could not find what I needed, my experiments with life have been put together for you so that you don't have to reinvent the wheel.

The book explores how to not only reverse but also to protect your immune system and prevent any further illness. Genetic predispositions can increase the risk of developing an autoimmune disease, so it's of paramount importance that you learn to reverse the illness and carry on a healthy self-care regimen so that you are passing on great health and being an excellent role model to your kids or grand kids.

> *You might wonder why a healthy self-care practice is so important after all. Here is where the larger and the most amazing piece that comes in to solve the autoimmune puzzle. It's the 'Epigenetics,' which determines how lifestyle changes and environmental factors largely influence the disease expression.*

Every single act, be it the foods you eat, your lifestyle stressors, the exercise activities you undertake or don't, your sleep patterns, and the impurities in the environment all play a crucial role in determining whether the genes are going to kick-start the disease in your body. Imagine genes as the match and the poor lifestyle choices as the frictions; these are going to create the prime conditions to ignite the fire. This was my moment of epiphany as I realized that my lifestyle choices can strongly influence the disease and bring it into remission. While genetics cannot be altered, we have greater influence over the influencers. The top 10 influencers are identified for you, so you can get started in adopting the MOTTOs into your day-to-day life and begin to experience The MOTTO Effect!

What's your MOTTO?

PART ONE
HELLO MOTO

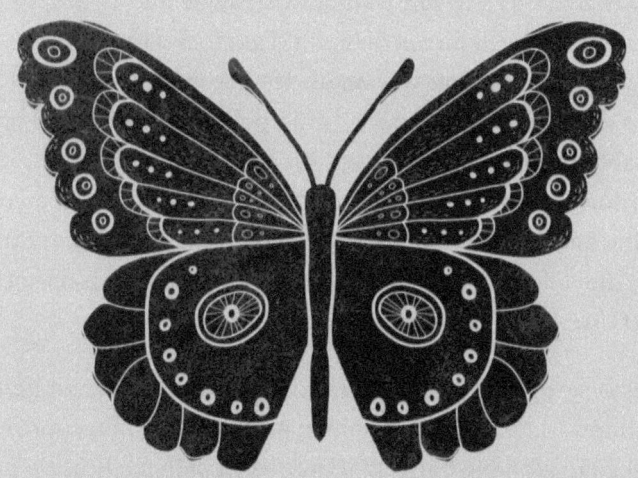

CHAPTER ONE

THE SUGARCANE MACHINE

It felt surreal to walk into the hospital for a random check with a big belly and to later come back home with a baby (and the big belly still there!) I was filled with euphoria each time I visualized moments of cuddles with my new little stranger, however, I was brought back to reality during my recovery, which made me feel down in the dumps. My emotions were up when I saw a healthy baby by my side, and rock bottom when I realized how battered my body felt. The terrible pain and struggle after the epidural wearing off hit me like a ton of bricks. I got to feel the contractions right where the incision was made. It took me few days to stand upright as the pain of the skin being pulled and stretched apart at the abdomen when I stood up was unbearable. Going through this period of pain and recovery made me realize I could overcome anything and showed me the strength and the power of motherhood. After all, most people say that delivering babies is one of the highest thresholds of pains one can endure.

I was slowly able to move around and continue with household chores while my sore abdomen was healing and recovering. I was asked to get a big bottle of ibuprofen, a pain medication from a wholesale club that contained 1000 capsules. Each day, my goal was to bring down the number of pain killers I was consuming, but during the first few weeks I had to gobble capsules every 2-4 hours. This meant I was taking in close to 2400mg of pain killers a day just to be able to do some of the bare minimum activities like walking around, laying on the bed or getting up to feed myself and the baby. If I ever happened to skip a dose, the intense burning and pain that felt like a sharp stabbing knife would return.

The next entry in my new mom life was the painful hemorrhoids - whoa! Just when I thought that nothing could be worse than a caesarean, this new pain proved otherwise. With the after effects of caesarean pain and the hemorrhoids added, it was a double-edged sword. Neither could I sit due to the shooting pain of the hemorrhoids, or lay down due to the pain in my abdomen. My bedside table was filled with medicines, as the painkillers were what kept me going during that period. With the intense sudden contractions in my uterus, every single part of my body was hurting. The greatest pleasure was dressing up my son in cute little baby outfits with matching socks and mittens and admiring him while I was pumping my milk. I loved to admire sleeping babies; they looked serene curled up on their tummy with their butt high up. Though my son was not old enough to sleep on his tummy yet, his occasional smiles during his naps would be heartwarming. Motherhood had days and nights of struggle but interspersed with moments, such as watching his post feed bliss that reassured me that I did all right.

I felt like I was running a whole dairy industry at my home, meticulously tracking the production, consumption, what was left out at the end of the day and did production increase - and what time of the day did it increase? After consuming fenugreek and oatmeal cookies did it increase? I was taking notes on all of the statistics. There was a lot of planning, strategy, tracking results and analyzing. I empathized with the cows a lot. How can cows produce so much? I was struggling for a few ounces. I felt like a cow, wandering aimlessly here and there, grazing on oatmeal cookies and producing.

Each passing day felt like the movie 'The Groundhog Day,' where the actor is caught in a time loop, repeatedly reliving all of the events of the day, every day. The never ending cycles of pump, feed, burp, put to sleep, swim through piles of dirty clothes to get to another room, clean bottles, eat and sleep myself, cook, stay awake all night listening to cries as my son was colicky, work full-time during the day - I had entered the zombie zone of my life! One night my sleep took over and I missed a pumping session totally unaware. Little did I realize that my over sleeping could cause the next wave of trouble; I ended up with mastitis, a painful infection of the breast tissue. Not a single part of my body was spared, I thought as I was given a dose of antibiotics. Mastitis feels like when you have a terrible flu, and I had recurring mastitis which left me totally wiped out. I had taken over sixty antibiotics by that stage, oblivious of the healthy bacteria I was destroying from my body. Heavy doses of antibiotics combined with the pain killers for the caesarean pain and suppositories for my bottom (which also was a frequent visitor) became the norm for me at one point in my life. I did the best to overcome the pain in the moment, but little did I realize how the medicines would add up to big health trouble later during my life.

I was grateful to have had a full-time work from home option and could take the initial few weeks of maternity leave. I enjoyed my work as a Brand Manager for a leading technology company. At that time, I received a job opportunity as a Brand Manager from a renowned pharmaceutical company whose main product was hemorrhoid medication, pop up in my LinkedIn feed. The universe has a great sense of humor I thought, I did know the brand inside out (pun intended) for sure! Although I did not look into the new opportunity that came up, it makes me laugh to this day thinking about the synchronicity.

Many moms talk about the love at first sight they had with their babies, for me it was gradual and the love came through an act. The act of caring, nurturing and making sure that my baby's needs were all met before mine, brought about the magical maternal feelings and a growing sense of responsibility and protection. Having a newborn can significantly change your perspective. I always saw my mother and father having a great sense of serenity raising kids for which I'm very grateful and appreciative of. I was nowhere close to parenting like them, rather **I was way more imperfect and worked beyond my super human capacity to give without much self-care.**

In India, there are sugarcane vendors on the roadside and it's fascinating to see how sugarcane juice is being made. The sugarcane is inserted in between two huge cylindrical rolling machines, it is crushed during this process and the juice is collected. To get the sweetest juice the sugarcane is inserted several times into the machine and only the remains of the sticks are left. The new mom demands felt similar to being crushed physically, mentally and emotionally, and I felt there was nothing left within me but, in the end, a happy baby is the sweetest juice I could ever experience.

CHAPTER TWO

THE REVOLVING DOOR

I continued to look pregnant and my body felt as though it were bursting at the seams, even 16 months after my son was born, so I really decided to play the part. I got pregnant again and was elated to have a baby girl. During the nesting stage of my pregnancy with my daughter, I became obsessed with tasks that weren't at the top of the list for what the baby might need. My energy levels really peaked during that time; I tried cooking several fancy dishes that were way beyond my imagination and usual culinary skills, which surprised my family because I was never into cooking something that takes a lot of time and effort. I cleaned all of the glass doors and windows on the outside of my home with a tissue and toothbrush in my hand, which surprises me even to this date (we have 17 of those!) and then had a pressure wash company do it all over again. Living in Arizona, dust storms were common, having the glass doors spick and span was always going to be the most futile effort and until this nesting stage, with its pronounced levels of energy, it would not have been considered for a moment.

Life seemed liked a rollercoaster of events. With two kids it was for sure twice the joy and twice the workload. You don't have to reinvent the wheel or buy new stuff. As second time parents we had a lot of things figured out, but it taught us some of the life's greatest lessons until this date - the value of time and multitasking. It was six months after my daughter was born, that I started to feel low most of the time. I lost weight quickly which I was excited about, all the post-baby body was lost and I was back to my pre-baby body shape. I had major trouble with getting a good night sleep; each morning when I woke up I would clear my hoarse throat for several hours and I felt as if I was losing my voice. I had foggy headaches every day which became the norm to me; I was way too fatigued and gradually lost interest in everything. My visit to the doctor revealed that I was hypothyroid with high numbers and was way beyond the recommended thyroid level range. When you are hypothyroid it means the thyroid gland cannot produce enough thyroid hormone to keep the body running normally. Some of my initial symptoms were fatigue, mood swings, lethargy and weight loss. With hypothyroid you tend to gain weight rather than lose it, so my symptoms did not exactly match hypothyroidism completely. I thought maybe it could be due to managing a two-and-a-half year old and a six-month old, plus working a full-time job too. I was immediately put on a medication to manage my thyroid levels.

The next few weeks I had frequent blood tests to monitor the level of thyroid medication and to make sure my levels were brought within the range; however, my symptoms seemed to worsen and not improve in any way. I felt that I had something more going on with me than the hypothyroidism.

> *I began to read and gain more knowledge about the thyroid; it's a butterfly shaped gland located at the base of your neck. This gland controls pretty much your entire body functioning – regulating your body temperature, the metabolic rate, heart and digestive function, muscle control, bone maintenance, brain development and mood. When the thyroid hormone production drops, the body's processes slow down leaving a person with multitude of symptoms.*

As the days progressed, my symptoms further worsened; waking up in the morning seemed to be the hardest part, and I felt groggy and hazy for the most part of the day. My body felt achy and thoroughly exhausted all the time even after a night's sleep. I would stay awake for several hours at night even though I longed for restful sleep, which never came easily to me. Even when I did sleep, my body never felt rejuvenated and I seemed to be stuck in a perpetual loop of low energy. It felt like I had to tremendously summon up everything in my energy reserve to accomplish even the simplest of tasks. I had to swim against the current relentlessly, day in and day out. My ideal day at that point was to stay in bed all day and do nothing, but of course, this was not an option. Mentally, just to think about all of the work that I had to do in any single day, made me feel miserable and defeated me before I had completed a single task. As a new mom, it's a fact that once you are out of bed, there would be an endless list of activities and chores to fulfil before you can go back to bed again.

After waking and dreading the day ahead, I would have a shower and then feel so fatigued that to even head to the closet to get my clothes felt an overwhelming task and I would want to lay down on the bed and just sleep. I was mostly bundled up in warm clothes and cozy socks as I felt cold most of the time, but would have sudden hot flashes and heart palpitations too. All the things that I once enjoyed no longer interested me, be it an activity, work, playing with kids, going out or reading - it was all too exhausting. When I did attempt to read, I found that my eyes were going over the same lines repeatedly and nothing made sense to me and the words were just a blurred mass on the page

All of a sudden my entire life seemed to have dulled down.

My doctor quickly suggested that I took an antidepressant in addition to my thyroid. Thankfully to this day I never started on one. Being hypothyroid mimics depression to a large extent, however there are some subtle differences that we need to understand.

More typical of Depression	More likely Hypothyroidism[1]
• Insomnia • Restlessness & inability to sit still • Feelings of worthlessness • Inappropriate guilt • Thoughts of death or suicide • Planning or attempting suicide	• Feeling chilled or overly sensitive to cold temperatures • Constipation • Muscle cramps or stiffness • Dry skin and hair • Hair loss • Hoarseness • Slowed heart rate

I developed a postpartum thyroiditis (PPT), where a previously normal thyroid gland becomes inflamed during the first year after child birth. In the United States, **postpartum thyroiditis occurs in approximately 5-10% of women[2]. This condition affects a small percentage of pregnant women, or about 3 in 100 to 2 in 25**[3]. Postpartum thyroiditis may first make your thyroid overactive (hyperthyroidism). This means it sends too much thyroid hormone out into the bloodstream. This can make parts of your body work too fast, but over time, the condition leads to an underactive thyroid (hypothyroidism). This means it doesn't make enough thyroid hormones and your body slows down. I was experiencing a wide range of symptoms from being hyper to hypo in a single day. It was similar to having two different bodies and experiences at the same time. I would feel warm at nights, to feeling cold during the day. Having anxiety, tremors in my hands and a racing heart beat in the morning to severe fatigue over the next few hours.

Some of the symptoms of hypothyroidism are: [4]

- Unexplained weight gain or trouble losing weight
- Fatigue
- Depression

- Hair loss and dry hair
- Muscle cramps
- Dry skin
- Goiter (swelling of thyroid gland)
- Brittle nails
- Slow heart rate
- Irregular period
- Sensitivity to cold
- Constipation
- Carpal tunnel syndrome

Some of the symptoms of hyperthyroidism are:
- Unexplained weight loss
- Feeling wired or anxious
- Racing heartbeat
- Shakiness
- Sweating spells
- Feeling hot, frequently
- Itchy red skin
- More frequent bowel movements than usual
- Fine hair and hair loss

Simple chores used to leave me confused – things like, did I turn on the dishwasher? Were the dishes washed or unwashed? I had to literally pick up a dish or two from the dishwasher to check if it was cleaned. At one of my doctor's appointment, the doctor casually asked when my daughter was born. I thought hard, racked my brains but could not for the life of me remember when she was born. "Well mommy-hood can make us have fish-like brains" she joked. I went back home that day still trying to recollect when my little girl was born, and by the time I went to bed that night I could not recall her birthdate. I had to actually look at my phone even to know the current year I was in, and had to work my way backwards to arrive at her birth year! I was appalled, my memory loss had worsened. It seemed to be more challenging to have to work with numbers than with words. On a separate note, my name Meena does mean fish; the comparison to fish-like brains statement did really have a lot of truth to it.

The memory loss continued for few more years. I even had trouble remembering my age. I used to use an app called the Wolfram Alpha to calculate my age. All you had to do was input your date of birth and calculate until it was the current date. Luckily I remembered when I was born. With my daughter, I had trouble recollecting her year of birth and had to go backwards, in my case I had to calculate from when I was born and go forward to know my age! Even 5-6 years after my son was born, I could not recollect many of the events that happened during that period which was a blur in my life.

Life seemed like a revolving door as I was visiting different doctors. I had the newborn checkups with the pediatrician for my daughter, wellness checkups for my son, dentists, eye examinations, post-delivery checkups with my gynecologist and later, I switched to my general practitioner for my thyroid. On each visit I would have my list of questions and concerns to be addressed between the three of us—myself, my son and my daughter. The visits also meant I needed to be aware of what was going on, making notes, doing a bit of research in advance and preparing my questions so I made good use of the time for both the doctor and I. After the visit, I had to make sure that I updated my notes. A lot of times I wished there was a doctor in the family, or dreamed of my husband being a doctor instead of an engineer - that would have helped us a lot. Or the least, if he could have studied medicine for a year or two and dropped off half way through before he continued on to becoming an engineer, I would joke. Walking in and out of doctor visits seemed like a normal daily activity for our family. I would walk through the clinic door carrying my daughter who was then six months old, which meant the trip was planned well in advance, making sure she had her bottles, that I had completed my pumping session, that we both were well fed – all whilst carrying huge bags. When heading out to work in the morning, my husband would ask which doctor are you visiting today? In the evening when he asked how the doctor's appointment was, I would ask which doctor he was referring to, being my absent-minded self.

I underwent several blood tests, and scans of my thyroid; then was recommended a chiropractor for the pains in my body, an acupuncturist for fatigue and headaches, and the list was continually growing. At one of my visits to the doctor, she asked how I was doing. I took the question quite literally and rattled off several symptoms that had become my norm. I did not realize it was a customary, plain "how are you doing" with only a short polite reply needed. The doctor was obviously not expecting to hear a rundown of my amassed symptoms. Because I was hurting all over, no crevice left untouched by a pain, ache or inflammation, with this one question I felt that someone really wanted to hear how I was doing and feeling. It was not a heartfelt connection I later realized. Every symptom I mentioned was keyed into the computer which churned out a list of medications based on the key word search. In my head I was screaming **"doctor you just heard 6 of my symptoms - I have 194 symptoms left!"** That day, I was determined not to leave without an answer. I could sense the doctor's impatience, she said, "You need to accept the new normal. You are a mom and life is never going to be the same as it was, neither is your body." That statement pierced directly through my heart, I knew I needed to move on and search for answers from a specialist. I could not accept this prognosis. The doctor dismissed me and I left her office with recommendations for the leading endocrinologists in the city.

CHAPTER THREE

THE DANCING SAMURAI'S

The recommendations were for three local top endocrinologists. After much research and analysis, I zeroed in on one. When I made my first call to the doctor's clinic I was shocked and dismayed to find out they were over-booked and that my first appointment would be after an eight month wait. My body was failing miserably and the severity of my symptoms increased - I knew I needed something right away or it would mean I'd have to do further research and finalize on a different doctor. So onto the next doctor it was, once again starting the research and reading reviews of patient's sharing lengthy experiences. Finalizing on a doctor is not all that easy, it was one of the hardest parts of all of this. When you are severely fatigued, reading through pages and pages of reviews and comments is not helpful and adds to the exhaustion. Brain fogged aka being brain dead, is really tough to manage - when what you're doing no longer makes sense to your body. You want to do something and follow it up with an action, but your brain says goodbye in the midst of it. Suddenly the primary command function is switched off and you're left with an aimless body trying to finish off what you started.

I somehow did manage to finish the research and decided to go with the second doctor. On making the initial outreach phone call, I was put on hold for 45 minutes. I felt that I had a unique condition, but it appeared that the endocrinologists were way too busy to even answer a call, which told me that I was not alone going through this. The research I did while the call was on hold for 45 minutes revealed that

> *The American Thyroid Association estimated 20 million Americans have some form of thyroid disease. Up to 60 percent of those with thyroid disease are unaware of their condition. Women are five to eight times more likely than men to have thyroid problems. One woman in eight will develop a thyroid disorder during her lifetime.*

My thoughts were interrupted when the receptionist on the other end said that the new patient wait would be 5 weeks but if there were any cancellations I would be called in earlier. It felt like a long few weeks wait. After four weeks of patiently waiting and doing more research to try and uncover some solutions, I had my first appointment with one of the city's leading endocrinologists. With all of my questions jotted down, I was eagerly looking forward to the visit.

The day arrived and after sitting for quite some time in the waiting room, I was called into the office. In less than five minutes I was dismissed from the office as the doctor suggested some additional tests and an ultrasound and once they had the results, there would be more to discuss during our next visit. After another week of waiting, the next appointment was due. The doctor said that I had something called Hashimoto's Thyroiditis. **"Thyroiditis" refers to "inflammation of the thyroid gland." Hashimoto's thyroiditis, also known as chronic lymphocytic thyroiditis, is the most common cause of hypothyroidism in the United States. It is an autoimmune disorder involving chronic inflammation of the thyroid**[1]**. Hashimoto's disease is an autoimmune disease, which means the body's immune system is attacking its own cells and organs. Normally, the immune system protects the body against infections caused by bacteria, viruses, and other harmful substances. In Hashimoto's disease, the immune system makes antibodies that attack and damage the thyroid. As a result, the thyroid**

gland becomes inflamed and hypothyroidism can develop[2].

With the doctor's voice becoming a fainter sound as he explained about how my own body was fighting against my thyroid, my mind overtook with its racing thoughts and images of Samurai's fighting against each other equipped with long swords. Why Samurai's? Maybe it was due to the Asian name Hashimoto's and the first image that sprang to my mind was the Samurai's. Hashimoto's thyroiditis was named after a Japanese physician who discovered it in 1912.

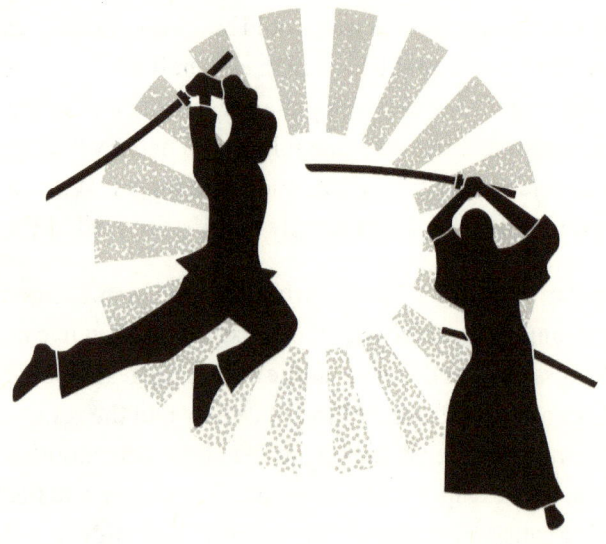

"Do you have any further questions?" the doctor's voice shook me back to my senses.

I did have a lot of questions this was all new to me; I was hearing about Hashimoto's for the very first time. The unique name and something so foreign made me feel alienated and like I was the only one to have this illness.

> *According to the American Autoimmune Related Diseases Association (AARDA), in the United States, autoimmune disease*

> *strikes one in five people, that's approximately 50 million Americans.*
>
> *Out of this, 75 percent affected are women, which is approximately 30 million. Autoimmune disease accounts for 90 percent of hypothyroidism, mostly due to Hashimoto's thyroiditis.*
>
> *Some of the data reveals that it's a public health crisis bigger than cancer and heart disease combined.*

Hashimoto's and hypothyroidism are not the same and cannot be used interchangeably. One of the leading causes of hypothyroidism is due to Hashimoto's. Hashimoto's is more of a progressive autoimmune condition, and unless the root causes are identified and resolved, the body would continue to attack the thyroid gland, which then eventually leads to thyroidism. I had lost a lot of time with my earlier doctor and the diagnosis of Hashimoto's had taken all of this valuable time. **If I look back at my illness journey, one of the biggest lessons I learnt is to know which lab tests are really needed to identify an autoimmune disorder, so that you do not lose time and health trying to figure this all out.** (Refer to the Lab Tests section)

What was next? I asked the doctor; he prescribed me some medication and said that we needed to continue to monitor the thyroid levels through blood tests - and the growing goiter (an abnormal enlargement of the butterfly-shaped gland below the Adam's apple) that I had on my throat with ultrasound tests, which is how it was discovered in the first place. I might have missed it all by myself. The growing lump had to be monitored to make sure the size was not increasing and if it did, then the next step suggested was surgery to remove the thyroid gland. I had a lot on my mind that day when I headed back home. I had gathered a lot of new information, and did some more research, as I wanted to know what exactly was happening to my body, but the fatigue caught up and

I had no choice but to retire to bed.

Waking up was getting harder as my sleep was disturbed by night sweats and racing thoughts. The next morning, I consumed the medication on an empty stomach, assuming that, boom, I would be well again - nothing seemed to change. With a severe pounding headache and having to clear my throat several times, I did notice that the hoarseness in my voice had increased. I sometimes seemed to even lose my voice completely for temporary periods of time, and talking at a louder volume was a strain. With having a toddler at home, getting into all kinds of mischief, it meant that most of the time my voice was strained and I could not keep up with the endless conversations that frequently required me to raise my voice. Eventually, the desire to converse was totally lost. I had lost interest in most things, and was sometimes taken over by such total mum guilt that I was not present with my kids during the most precious time of their lives. The top symptoms that really screamed so loudly at my body were - fatigue, hoarseness, body pains, headaches, anxiety, lack of interest, brain fog, terrible hair loss, but there were a ton of other symptoms that were not even brought to question by the doctors.

> *There was nothing left inside of my head thanks to the brain fog and memory loss or on the outside of my head due to severe hair loss.*

I was engulfed in my own misery and I was clearly drowning. We all love to be that super woman who can prove that we can take care of the family, have the chores managed to a tee, work a full-time job and remain sane. I was on the hamster wheel, literally running around in circles making no progress. Feeling exhausted, overwhelmed and no matter what I achieved, there was always more to do; little ones relying on me to be taken care of, unmet needs, gaps to fill, always more, more…

Nothing that I said or did made sense to me or to my family members. The stress of working and taking care of my family was transforming me into a raging monster; little things would cause me a lot of irritation and anger and I did not have any control over my thoughts or my feelings. I clearly remember when my parents were visiting me from India, the day they were leaving, I let loose my rage. Words left my mouth and flew like missiles; they left feeling dejected and this feeling continued for their entire journey home during their 24 hours flight back to India. I felt I had become a person whom I never wanted to be; this was totally not me – I was unrecognizable. My expression of anger was not welcomed by anyone in the family. As women, we live in a world where every role you play as daughter, as mom, as wife or as daughter-in-law, you are expected to be serving, caring, nurturing and not really show your true self. While they were visiting, there was a social event that I wanted to skip for the sake of my wellbeing - I needed a piece of my life back and some quietness. Dressing up, being nice and making a social appearance was not what my heart wanted. My heart pleaded for more of me-time, time of solitude. My family was shocked by my behavior. They were so upset and they said that they did not have the interest to attend the event any longer without me. "I'd changed a lot. Why could I not make it? What were the others going to think about me?" Complex questions were raised, but they forgot to consider what I was thinking or feeling and how unwell I felt. I finally gave in and ended up going to the event to make peace with my family. In those moments I questioned myself, and my small world made up of the people whom I loved the most, were the ones who were shown the worst side of me. Somewhere along the way I was losing connection with myself and with others.

When you're in pain deep within and hurting, everything externally can be a trigger. I needed to stop the snap circuit.

The more pain within → more triggers → more arguments → regret of my self-expression → suppression → more deep seated pain

I began to stop expressing my emotions - anger, rage, irritation, hurt, misery; I bottled up everything within me. My true expressions caused more chaos and disharmony at home. Speaking the truth led to more disruption and the impact that it created was a lot harder to resolve. Self-expression was shunned so I went silent. To the outside world, they thought I was doing well, but my internal world had already been crushed beyond reason. Any thoughts or emotions I had during this journey were all pushed down and festered within me. I did what I had to do to be the mother, daughter, wife, daughter-in-law and an employee.

For a year, getting out of bed was hard, but I made sure my kids were comfortable in their beds and slept well. Having a shower was hard, but I gave nice warm oil massages to my kids before their showers. Carrying myself around was hard, but I carried two toddlers for many months. I cooked, cleaned, did laundry, and worked a full-time job, managed a two and half year old and a six month old. I did well in the world's eye, but my personal struggle was overwhelming. For several months my only thought was "I wish someone cared for me and that I had more support." I counted my small victories along the way, when things were hard I did it anyway because with each pain that one endures, you get stronger. I kept asking what could be worse than caesarean pain? What could be worse than hemorrhoids? That kept me going through life with more courage and dignity.

My visits to the endocrinologist continued, my medication levels were being modified and my goiter monitored. My goiter had become stable at one point and there was no further growth which meant a surgery was ruled out. I was relieved; never did I ever want to remove my thyroid. I was experiencing a rollercoaster of symptoms thrust between being hyper to hypothyroid and I was back at being hyperthyroid due to over medication. Frequent visits to the endocrinologists led to nowhere. Only my medication levels were being monitored but the overall symptoms continued to exist. The time arrived that I felt I needed to look beyond western medicines.

The search began.

END OF PART ONE
CHECK-IN

1. How are you feeling today?
___

2. What symptoms are you experiencing physically, mentally and emotionally? Start all the way from the top of your head and do a check-in with each part of your body all the way to your feet. Nothing is too small not to consider. Take notes and keep track. (Refer to the Symptom Checker.)
___

3. How do you feel about your life in general? Do you feel in control / overwhelmed in any area of your life? (Health, Beauty, Kids, Relationship, Spouse, Finance, Home, Job)
___

4. Do you have someone to support you through this journey? Who can you reach out to? (Good medical practitioner / Naturopath / Friend)
___

SYMPTOM CHECKER

Here is the list of my symptoms I had experienced in varying degrees.

HEAD

- [ ] headaches
- [ ] faintness / dizziness
- [ ] racing thoughts
- [ ] hair fall
- [ ] greying

MIND

- [ ] brain fog
- [ ] poor memory
- [ ] poor overall mind and body coordination
- [ ] difficulty making decisions
- [ ] attention deficit and learning issues

EYES, NOSE AND EARS

- [ ] blurred vision
- [ ] dark circles
- [ ] nasal congestion
- [ ] loss of smell
- [ ] ringing in ears
- [ ] ears feel always blocked

MOUTH/THROAT

☐ frequent throat clearing
☐ sore throat
☐ hoarseness / losing voice
☐ canker sores
☐ loss of taste
☐ gum disease –periodontal disease
☐ tongue that does not look pink and healthy – it could be coated white

HEART

☐ palpitations
☐ shortness of breath

SKIN

☐ hives
☐ acne
☐ excessive sweating
☐ hot flushes
☐ feeling cold or warm
☐ pigmentation
☐ dryness
☐ dullness
☐ looking aged

WEIGHT

- ☐ weight gain
- ☐ weight loss
- ☐ food cravings especially salty foods and carbs
- ☐ swelling/water retention in the body
- ☐ compulsive mood based eating

DIGESTION

- ☐ nausea
- ☐ vomiting
- ☐ constipation
- ☐ haemorrhoids
- ☐ bloating
- ☐ uneasiness after eating
- ☐ heartburn/indigestion
- ☐ stomach cramps

EMOTIONS

- ☐ anxiety
- ☐ depression
- ☐ mood swings
- ☐ tremors/shakiness
- ☐ irritability
- ☐ getting hangry with eating delays

BODY, JOINTS AND MUSCLES:

- ☐ joint pains in the morning
- ☐ carpal tunnel on right wrist
- ☐ muscle weakness
- ☐ neck and back pain
- ☐ leg cramps
- ☐ restless leg syndrome
- ☐ varicose veins
- ☐ fatigue
- ☐ lethargy
- ☐ restlessness

PART TWO
STUMBLING ONTO MOTTO'S

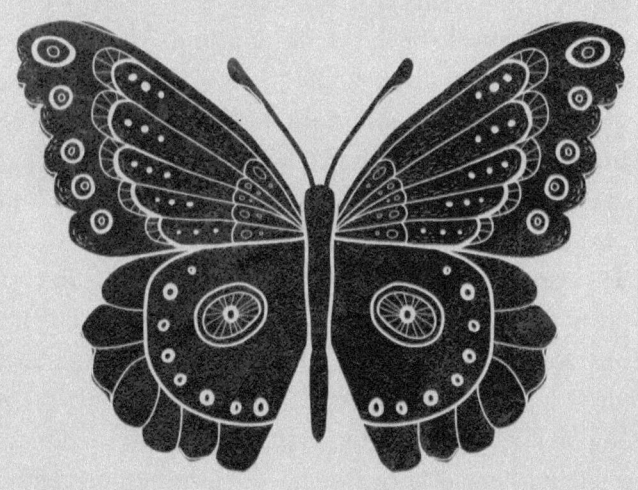

CHAPTER FOUR

GOOGLE GUIDED

An exhausting year went by with absolutely no difference in the way that I felt or any improvement in my symptoms. In fact, the number of symptoms increased and few of the long term ones worsened. I read somewhere that pain lets you know you're alive - I felt so alive! In the mornings when I woke up, my joints would crack and pop so much that my family used to wake up. My joint cracks were their morning alarm. There was significant achiness and stiffness in my joints that I noticed as soon as I woke up, which would eventually be fine as the day progressed. However, I had nagging wrist pain throughout the day which worsened and I could not use the laptop or write much in the end. I wore the carpal tunnel braces for several months. I noticed my hair was greying out a lot and my hair loss was terrible - I was dismayed by the clumps of hair that came out after a shower. I had thick hair and the thinning was so drastic that I lost nearly 60% of my hair. It was ironic that none of the hairs that fell out were those naughty grey hairs! I felt frustrated as there was no remedy to regain the lost hair. . Every time I looked in the mirror it brought about more sadness. For a long time, I tied my hair up in the hope that it would reduce the hair fall but that never really helped. I later began to embrace a shorter hairdo to make up for the loss.

I hoped to recover by just taking the thyroid medication Synthroid that I was prescribed. Like millions of people who suffer with this condition, that's the most common recommendation from conventional treatment and to continue to be on medication forever. I was under medicated, then over medicated and then termed as normal thyroid levels based on my blood work results but I was nowhere close to good health. I fluctuated between low and high levels for a while until my levels could stabilize. That was one of the most erratic periods in my life, I had no control over my mind or body which was terrifying. On hypothyroid days (when the thyroid levels were low) I had zero interest in activities, or even having a conversation with anyone, all I wanted to do was to be left alone. It felt like I was tied to a rock and I had a struggle to perform every single activity. On hyperthyroid days (when the thyroid levels were high) it would be a hyper day with palpitations, anxiety, excessive sweating, feeling warm, excessive hunger, racing thoughts, severe headaches that would last all day, and being fidgety. All the hyper activity would also cause excessive fatigue but mentally nothing would seem to calm me down. I would experience a combination of hypo and hyper symptoms all in one day. It was the most difficult phase to comprehend what I was experiencing for myself, so there was no way I could have explained this to others in my family back then and the only one to help out would be my doctor, or so I thought.

> *Unfortunately, I realized that I was trying to climb the ladder of optimal health that was leaning against the wrong wall.*

If other symptoms popped up, then different medications were prescribed and ultimately the root cause was ignored and the symptoms were focused on. The underlying imbalances and inflammations were not targeted. None of this enlightenment came to me during my earlier days of struggle. I only knew that I was not feeling better and I needed to look at other alternatives out of sheer desperation.

Constant blood tests and long wait times at the doctors, only to be called into the office, then barely getting to spend ten minutes with the doctor made me highly frustrated. I would have waited for a few weeks to get that appointment, hoping to make some progress in my recovery and ultimately each time it would turn out to be the same old story of needing yet more tests, more reports which lead to more medical bills. The doctor always seemed rushed and would storm into the room with his assistant, where I would have waited for over thirty minutes, only to go over the previous report quickly, request for me to go in for further tests and then turn around and walk out. There would have been no real conversation, which disappointed me and I was truly fed up with the entire process. Sometimes the dosage was adjusted then later on when it was normalized as per the records, the visits made me realize there was little value for my time. I feared to even blurt out symptoms after a few visits, since I knew what was coming – anti-depressants, pain medications, sleeping pills, or more tests. I was convinced during some of these discussions with the doctor that it was a lifelong condition and there was no complete recovery from it. I was also told that if one has an autoimmune condition they would be prone to several other types of autoimmune disorders or even a heart condition later on in life. The doctor remarked that it could also be due to aging but I was only in my early thirties! **However, I do know the severity of avoiding any medication approach. Untreated, thyroid disorders can lead to many complications which can include heart problems, nerve injury, and infertility or even be fatal.** If you are pregnant and have an untreated thyroid disorder, your child may have a higher risk of birth defects than babies born to healthy mothers.

Hashimoto's experience was similar to driving through a traffic jam in India. Driving on Indian roads would feel like riding on a bumper car - out of nowhere there would be vehicles coming at you from different directions, sometimes bumping into you, or someone on a bicycle trying to elbow his way through and you are scared and hope he doesn't scratch your precious car; pedestrians sporadically crossing; even cows or dogs strolling in between the traffic.

Sometimes you would be stuck in traffic for eternity and notice a tea vendor, calm and collected, trying to sell tea to the drivers who were his captive market. Watching the tea vendor is a class act; he would approach the cars quickly and from what seems nowhere and weave through the traffic so swiftly before shoving the tea cup right in front of your face. You might have been unaware and may have never intended on having tea, but you end up drinking it because it's directly in front of your face and before you realize the reality of the situation, he's got the money and has moved out and onto the next unsuspecting customer. When the drama is over you notice that the traffic jam has not moved an inch and you're still stuck in the same place where you were before.

This disorder felt the same way, you have hundreds of symptoms jumping out of nowhere from different areas of your body; you are caught unaware and then left stuck with these symptoms. You have the doctor giving the medications amidst all of the body chaos - similar to the tea vendor. Having the tea or the medication in this instance, is not really addressing the core issue (the traffic) or treating the cause of symptoms. A year had passed by, I wondered what had I done all this while; I had the medications and umpteen tests but was stuck in life's traffic jam.

I was taking my medications dutifully, never missing a dose; I would have it first thing in the morning on an empty stomach and wait for an hour before I had my breakfast. Having coffee immediately after taking the thyroid medication reduces the effectiveness of it, so it's important to wait for at least an hour. I don't recollect what time I used to wake up then, but nowadays I keep my alarm set for 4am then just rollover, reach out to my bedside, take the medication and go back to sleep to wake up at 5am (I'm sure I would have never woken up at 5am then). This way I get the minimum one hour wait time, a little more sleep and get to wake up to my freshly brewed coffee. During the day, I could hardly wait until my afternoon nap. Luckily, I used to work on east coast time zone so I used to start my work early, end it early and then take a nap. I read that Nikola Tesla, the inventor of alternating-current (AC) electric system used to sleep only for 2-3 hours every night. I felt guilty when I read that, I used to nap for 2-3 hours in the afternoon!

I knew I had to find an alternative but was not sure if it would be another doctor or if there were other specialists who could help me. My general practitioner had recommended acupuncture during one of my visits. When I was reading up about acupuncture I came across alternative medicine related searches which finally led me to naturopaths. I had very limited awareness about naturopaths or if they could treat this illness. When there are no answers for problems in life, there's always google. Google is like a mirror reflecting your own thoughts so nowhere did I ask for how worse would one feel with Hashimoto's - I knew the answer for that. I was looking for "what next" instead of "why me?" There was no time for self-pity at this stage in life, my only mission was to recover and to take care of my kids for whom I had to heal as quickly as possible, I felt that time was running out and I had already wasted far too long. I felt convinced that there might be someone who could help me out with this illness and my job was to find that person. This really helped me to move on in this stage. If I had sat down searching for "why me", then I'm sure there would be pages and pages of proven research that there was no recovery from this which would not have helped me in any way. Never taking a 'no' for the final answer kept me going tenaciously.

Even though this illness was common, the solutions were not clearly laid out, nor at least within my reach. **Each individual can be unique in their symptoms ranging along a wide spectrum of all to none, to many, to something totally different, which made it difficult with the conventional approach to think of solutions**

totally out of the box and have a customized treatment for the patients instead of following a rigid pill-only approach.

Searching for a naturopath, I realized there were many to my surprise, but once again choosing the right one meant more research. I had to choose someone that specialized in autoimmune illnesses. I actually spent more time searching for a Naturopath than I did choosing my life partner. Also, I was not sure what the method of treatment might be so I had a dose of mild skepticism. Most practices also insisted on retaking several tests which I was not in favor of. I had already gone through this loop of one test after another and was really looking for something that might help me to recover faster. I was not sure if this was the right route, but was willing to give it a try. There was nothing left to lose; if this approach did not work I would stay where I was. If it worked then I could be on my road to recovery.

And so, my next step in my path ahead was with the naturopath.

CHAPTER FIVE
EXPANSIVE AWARENESS

I waited eagerly at the Naturopath's office, part of me feeling a sense of deja vu at having been in this situation before. I was not sure what to expect with the new doctor and felt a fair amount of apprehension. My mind raced and I felt preoccupied, as the only thing I had gained in my year-long visits with my earlier doctors was a hefty medical bill. Naturopaths are typically not covered by insurance, so I hoped and put faith in the fact that I had made the right decision. The last thing I wanted was for my health treatments to become a financial burden to my family. I would rather invest the money for my children's future than to spend it on myself, unless it made me well again. After a warm welcome at the front desk I was asked to fill out a few pages, it actually seemed a lot more than what I had typically done anywhere else. Health and family histories were the customary details. Some sections required spending a lot of time to answer the depth of the questions – the degree of stress in my life, to list different events that had taken place and any recent changes in my life, my current lifestyle, there was an entire page on fatigue plus an entire page on digestion, mental and emotional health. Some of these questions are typically not asked at a doctor's office. I took a long time to respond to these questions and was glad that I had arrived early; it felt like for the first time in my life I actually sat down to take a good honest look at my life and reflect. My life had zoomed past me so fast that this quiet time, sitting with these questions and my thoughts felt blissful. There was no rush, no pressure and I was asked to take more time if needed.

I was greeted with a big warm smile by the Naturopathic Doctor (ND). His sense of calmness and poise instantly made me feel more at ease. "How are you doing?" he asked sincerely. I had a paragraph length of an answer in my mind, but I cut it short to a one-word reply of "good." That was what the past experience at the doctor's office had taught me.

"Well, tell me more" he said which took me by surprise.

I made myself a lot more comfortable on the couch and sat back and opened up - we talked for two hours at length and in depth! At the end of the discussion, not only did I feel genuinely hopeful that I could recover, I also had made the first real connection with a doctor in my life. It was heartfelt; I could sense the genuine care he held. I'm an introvert who loves deep, genuine, heartfelt conversations. **During the initial struggle with Hashimoto's, I feel as long as you have the quality support you can get through life in that state.** You only need someone who can sit with you, hold the space and actively hear you as you empty your heart and mind. Sadly, since we are so messed up physically, mentally and emotionally, the words that come out hardly make much sense. During that appointment, we went over most of the answers in the form I had filled out and the ND had more questions to help him understand my situation better.

ND's are used to listening to long lists of symptoms. It is totally normal to experience over 200+ symptoms I was told, after all, the thyroid regulates all of the activities in your body. When the base controller is out, different parts of the body send out the emergency warnings. That day I felt I had made more progress with understanding this illness than I ever had in any of the doctor's visits during the past twelve months.

The first step to healing for me came when I realized there was someone who was able to listen to me which gave me the validation to know that what I was experiencing was normal. There were times when I would question myself and doubt as to how I could experience so many symptoms, to the extent that there was a complete shift in my true identity as a person. The discussions not only probed into what was happening in my life, but also what really mattered to me in my life which is another step towards making that real connection between the physician and the patient. With my previous endocrinologist, there was always a time bomb and dollar signs adding up that were constantly ticking with each visit. The constant reminding that a surgery may be necessary to remove the thyroid during repeated visits, only made me feel the future was bleak with little choice, it left me feeling powerless. With my ND, there was deep trust and belief and it was a partnership where we were jointly working towards a recovery. After recommending an approach or a supplementation, there was always constant checks to make sure I felt good and there were no adverse symptoms which was reassuring (Refer to the Lab Tests and Medications section).

During one of my visits, my ND inquired as to how my fatigue levels were and asked if I might have any vague idea on when I was more tired - was it in the mornings or the evenings? I said yes, I knew it was in the mornings and to be precise between 9 and 11am – as that was the time I wanted to really hit the bed. He was amazed; he said not many patients were able to distinguish the exact time. When you're fatigued for several years, it's hard to be aware of when you specifically hit the peak fatigue period. It's rather like picking a needle out of the haystack. He quickly brought out a multi colored chart that had different markings on it. Traditional Chinese Medicine (TCM) discovered a body clock that can help one understand the way that energy moves through our bodies to restore and activate different functions of the organs.

TRADITIONAL CHINESE MEDICINE CLOCK

Heart (11 A.M to 1 P.M)
Eat lunch and socialize!

Small Intestine (1 P.M to 3 P.M)
Solve your problems and get organized!

Spleen (9 A.M to 11 A.M)
Work and be active!

Bladder (3 P.M to 5 P.M)
Work, study and drink tea!

Stomach (7 A.M to 9 A.M)
Eat breakfast!

Kidneys (5 P.M to 7 P.M)
Eat dinner and restore your energy!

Large Intestine (5 A.M to 7 A.M)
Wake up and drink water!

Pericardium (7 P.M to 9 P.M)
Intimacy and procreation!

Lungs (3 A.M to 5 A.M)
Sleep soundly!

Triple Warmer (9 P.M to 11 P.M)
Chill out, relax and read!

Liver (1 A.M to 3 A.M)
Deep resting and dreaming!

Gallbladder (11 P.M to 1 A.M)
Sleep and regenerate!

EXPANSIVE AWARENESS

"Chinese Medicine's 24 hour body clock is divided into 12 segments consisting of two hours per segment. In each of these segments, our Qi (vital life force or known as the "prana") moves through the body, landing in a specific organ meridian. During sleep, Qi is drawn inward to restore the body. This phase is completed between 1 and 3 A.M, when the blood is cleansed by the liver and the body performs several other functions to ensure the Qi is ready to move out of the body again. When one organ is at its peak energy, the organ at the opposite side of the clock, 12 hours away, is at its lowest function. So in my case, my body's energy was affected by the 9-11pm organs which were 12 hours away and at their lowest function. The organs I'm referring to were my thyroid and adrenals which it states as responsible for energy, transfer, temperature and metabolism. So I wanted my body to function as if it were the 9-11am level of working and be active, whereas it was responding to the 9-11pm zone of chilling out and relaxed! I was mind blown - this was way too accurate in my case.

Triple Warmer is the meridian that controls our fight, flight or freeze response. According to Donna Eden, author of Energy Medicine, the triple warmer impacts the immune system and our ability to manage stress. At a psychological level the triple warmer meridian is connected to the throat. The throat center is governed by sound, and is where we speak what we feel is true for ourselves - it is the center for self-expression. When we feel we are "acting like someone else" then we are not in tune with our true self. When we speak against our feelings we are blocked. The throat is where we swallow – at the physical level it is food, at the psychological level those are the thoughts that we later manifest[3]. In ancient India the chakra system was discovered similar to the TCM; **the throat chakra or known as Visuddha in Sanskrit is connected to the way in which we express life with authenticity.** When the throat chakra is blocked, one could experience physical symptoms, like a frequent sore throat or laryngitis – but perhaps more significantly, it could leave you struggling to express your inner truth, or unable to communicate with confidence and honesty.

In medical terms it means the adrenals and the thyroid are interrelated. The thyroid is located at the base of the neck and it produces the thyroid hormone responsible for maintaining the body's metabolism. The adrenals are located on top of the kidneys that produce stress hormones (epinephrine, norepinephrine, and cortisol), some sex hormones, and mineralocorticoids, which regulate fluid balance and blood pressure. Prolonged or intense stress can raise the cortisol levels which can lead to adrenal fatigue due to overworking of the adrenal gland. The adrenal glands are unable to keep up with the constant demand for flight or fight arousal. Excess cortisol also inhibits the thyroid from making more thyroid hormones or vice versa, as when the cortisol levels are low, the thyroid levels are shown to increase. Adequate cortisol levels are needed to have a well-functioning thyroid system. I realized my thyroid symptoms were not merely a thyroid problem, my cortisol levels needed to be stable. Hence the cortisol imbalance could not be corrected by just taking the thyroid medications; I also had to support my cortisol levels. That was one of the reasons why even though my blood reports showed normal levels and was well within the thyroid range, I was no way close to recovery. It was somewhat of a breakthrough moment for me.

Connecting the dots, I could finally see clearly that my stress levels and exhaustion, which peaked after my son was born, continued to remain at that level, and worse, for a few years and caused my body to completely shut down after my daughter was born. My body had run 200mph after my son was born, as I continued to run the beaten up car with a low battery, a poor engine and bad fuel and it ultimately came to a grinding halt. In the early mornings, the automatic start failed and I had to go for the self-start mode which lasted only for a few hours. My spluttering car was sending out signals all throughout the day to 'check the engine' which I failed to notice. Added to this was my perfectionism which was the perfect recipe for disaster. I worked on being the super mom and no less, cooking up baby foods from scratch, tried hard to maintain a clean home, determinedly work my way to the top in my career yet I kept falling short of my own set high standards and the never ending to-do lists that kept me going in that cycle.

Working from home involved taking on a lot of calls and constantly being on back to back online meetings. My typical day would start with a 7am call, so I would be busy on the phone call, have the laptop on the kitchen table, multi-tasking to madness whilst fixing breakfast on one side of the kitchen and being available as an employee on the other side of the room. Most times the call would last for up to two hours, which meant I would have never had time for a single word or a kind-hearted good bye to my husband each morning. I was making sure the task of having the family ready for the day and fed was taken care of, but deep hearted conversations were masked by the busyness of my work and fell by the wayside. All day I would work to exhaustion, it was go, go, go and even my lunch used to be rushed over meetings and I would not have time to clear up the kitchen. By the time my family was back home in the evening, I was depleted of my energy to care for them, the kitchen would be in a messy disaster with dishes left over since breakfast so then I would focus on restoring order to the home rather than focusing on them. Working from home also meant frequent traveling, which I had to avoid several times due to my failing health and taking care of kids. When my co-workers were able to travel and I was the only one who had stayed back, it did not reflect well as per corporate terms, as out of sight meant out of mind when it came to promotions. I had to take up marketing projects and work closely with the office of the CEO. It meant time pressured projects with the highest attention to details and very strict deadlines. I had to be present on chat, phone call or available for a meeting at any hour during the day. I could not keep up with the intense work load and would end up working late hours. I knew my body was failing, I was exhausted beyond means and I knew the answer was to take a break from my job, but I could not really zero in on what it was that made me not want to accept that my body desperately needed to stop and require restoration way earlier than I intended to.

Not only did I get to understand what was happening within my body, the statement that the ND made, that not many people are aware of when exactly they get tired, gave me a spark of hope on self-awareness – which really was the beginning of this journey. This was the first step towards much greater consciousness that was to follow. **I kept track of my fatigue levels, made notes on how my body reacted to certain foods, how I felt before and after food, how the medication changes made me feel and moved to my emotional awareness of when did I get more frustrated or agitated. What were the triggers in my life? Were those self-imposed?** I worked on lowering my expectations and standards in a way that was right for me. All of this did not happen in a single day, it was gradual but nevertheless, I began to slowly start seeing the results. After the early morning 7am call I would have previously gulped down a big cup of coffee loaded with sugar that fueled my adrenaline for an hour or two. As soon as the call ended I came back to my senses and realized that what I really wanted to do was crash on the couch, not being able to distinguish between fatigue and hunger, delayed my breakfast which would cause tremors in my body. I would fix a breakfast in hurry and shove it down my throat so as not to be late for the next meeting.

> *The first step towards any healing process is to pause and get in touch with your body, mind and soul. We are constantly on the play mode skipping past interruptions. Always doing and not being.*

It's not easy in our modern fast paced world but it can be achieved. With consciousness we can fix it one step at a time. If you feel you are in this stage, the pointers below would help you to progress to the next stage.

- Find someone to talk to and support you throughout this journey.

- If you don't already have one, then find a good holistic medical practitioner, this might be hard to find but worth the effort. You may use local social media channels and community networks to identify one.

- Wherever you are, whatever you are doing, just stop. Pause and listen to your body. Everything else can wait. Your body has the biggest clear message for you when you are ready to hear it!

LAB TESTS AND MEDICATIONS

Here are the essential tests to take to know a lot more about your current health.

The only test that is typically done is the Thyroid Stimulating Hormone (TSH) and maybe T4 levels (which determines the concentration of thyroid hormone in your blood). Since I had received only these tests for a long time, the diagnosis of Hashimoto's did not come until much later on.

Make sure you receive the below tests.

1. Full Thyroid Panel: which includes TSH, Free T4, Free T3, Reverse T3, Thyroid Peroxidase antibodies (TPO) and Thyroglobulin antibodies (TG). *(The antibodies test will show the autoimmune levels currently present in your body. Working on these levels is the first step towards recovery.)*

2. Food Allergy / Sensitivity Test

3. Gut infections: Bacterial, Fungal and Parasitic infections can be tested to identify gut infections.

4. Vitamin B12 levels, Vitamin D levels, Iron Folate levels.

Right Medication

- T4 medication: I was on Levothyroxine (a T4 medication), which is the most largely prescribed one. Later I switched to Synthroid (a brand name version of the same T4 medication). There are several synthetic T4 hormone medications Levo-T, Levothyroxine, Novothyrox, Synthroid, Unithroid.

- T3 medication: the real game changer for me in terms of my energy levels when I added T3 along with my T4 medication. Liothyronine is the most largely prescribed one and the branded version is Cytomel or Triostat.

- T1, T2, T3 and T4: There are Natural Desiccated Thyroid (NDT) medication options which have a combination of T4 as well as T3, T1 and T2 that are available only through compounded pharmacy. These medications are derived from the thyroid gland of pigs and are considered as bio identical hormones. Several patients have seen great improvements with these medications. Armor, Nature-Throid, WP Thyroid all are NDT medications. Personally I had not used any of these.

Once the autoimmune attacks reduce and then stop, the thyroid can heal by itself and some patients can successfully even wean off of thyroid medications with the advice of the doctor!

CHAPTER SIX

INTENTIONALLY ME

I sat down and prioritized my list of symptoms and had it narrowed down to the top five symptoms that I needed to work on the most. Living with a multitude of symptoms, from head to toe, it is hard to prioritize, nevertheless, I categorized my symptoms so it seemed more achievable. Here were my top 5 most troublesome symptoms back then.

1. Fatigue

2. Pains – joints, wrist, neck, headaches, muscle pain

3. Digestion issues - bloating, uneasiness after eating, hemorrhoids, constipation

4. Emotional/mental - brain fog, memory loss, sluggishness, moody, irritable, depressed

5. Skin and hair - severe hair loss, greying hair, skin dullness, looking aged

The clear winner from the list was my fatigue. During one of my visits with the ND, he asked what were some of my other concerns with my skin? I said, "Doctor, if I can get my energy back, I can focus on my beautification goals and get myself back on track in that area of life". I was determined to get my energy levels back more than anything. I started reading about regaining energy; my quest for energy led me to a much greater path that I could never have imagined when I first got started on it. I searched for what made me feel energetic and what really sapped my energy. I realized energy is everything and in everything. I felt it was a key to unlocking a big secret in my life. I got engrossed in the topic of energy and read about it a lot during my journey.

I worked with my ND to fix my thyroid and adrenal health aspects. I knew I was in good hands with the medical aspect. My personal commitment began first in the area of time management. With little ones, a job and minimal energy levels I had to become more efficient and compartmentalize my time. **I had just a few blocks of time during the day to finish up work as I knew my battery would run low quickly. I undertook activities based on the level of intensity and focus it required and on the specific times I knew my attention span was good.** Every night before hitting bed, I had my next day's tasks all written down in advance, so mentally I was training my mind to stay alert and focus on finishing up the tasks on hand. I knew I had a small window of time open, so I remained focused on just that one activity during that period of time, this helped me to store up my energy since it was not diffused by multi-tasking for longer periods of time. This gave me a boost of energy and once I had completed my task I moved onto the next one with more zest. My weakness was becoming my biggest strength. I realigned my priorities to what mattered most. Mundane tasks or chores like laundry and dishes that required no mental alertness, I moved to during my slump times or right before bed time. I focused on what I had to accomplish each day, one day at a time and I divided my tasks morning to evening. The first set of tasks was before lunch and then the next set of tasks were after lunch and nap. After lunch was my slump time where I used to feel most zoned out. Then once again, I would take up high priority tasks right after my afternoon nap when I was most energized. Each day and each hour I had my mental battery running at the background similar to a cell phone displaying the battery levels on the surface. Needing to complete as much as possible within those specific buckets of time encouraged me to learn to set my boundaries. I always had a little bit of buffer and I learnt to also listen to my body's needs. Some days I could not accomplish much even though I was mentally prepared the previous day. So this meant what was not done in the morning would then move to the evening to-do's. I was getting good at prioritizing; not just that, I was significantly improving at estimating how long each task would take and I could plan my day accordingly. It seemed like a mini game with my brain to see if my estimated time met the actual time taken to accomplish and I enjoyed it.

> *This was also the beginning to building mental resilience; I was slowly growing my mental muscle to accomplish tasks irrespective of how my body was functioning then.*

When I look back I realize this is what living in the moment meant. My memory was still not that great which meant I had to focus more intently and reread a lot, for which I had to factor in more time. I also had to write everything down, else it disappeared from my memory bank. The good thing was that I forgot all that needed to be forgotten. It was the universe's way of emptying my cup so it could be filled only with goodness. I see or read about how women can always remember all the nitpicky things from months ago and bring it all up back up to the surface during fights, I'm fortunate to have had poor memory as we never had any of the flash backs making their entry into our fights - we stayed in the present moment even during fights!

During that time my husband and I also decided to leave our kids at a day care. For most moms I know that can be a nerve-wracking experience to leave their kids elsewhere and wonder how they are doing the entire day. We were grateful to find a nice day care close to our home. The first day when I went to drop off my kids, the owner held my hand and asked me not to worry and said I could check on my kids anytime by calling her as she knew how hard it can be and heart breaking. She had the full blown emotions, much more than I did. I dropped off my kids, came back to my car, and gave a big emphatic smile. For the first time, I was by myself. I felt liberated and the feeling of freedom and peace set in. I played music in my car all the way back home that day. With all honesty, I enjoyed my personal me time which had been long overdue. The kids had a great time there and it worked out brilliantly for all of us in the long run. The constant pressure to prepare food, feed the kids, put them to nap, bathe them, clear up the kitchen after their feeds, diaper changes, was a whole lot of work that had just evaporated. Every important piece of work that needed to be done depended on their nap time and the stress of waiting for the opportune moment to handle tasks was removed out of my life.

After a few months, I made the next important decision in my life to leave my job. It was a double whammy as we had our kids in the day care which meant paying for those expenses and also losing a full time paycheck each month. I felt that if I had my kids in the daycare, my situation would improve, but I realized I was completely exhausted with my full-time job on my plate too.

> *All of the early signs my body was giving me were disguised with the busyness of my life.*

I could not pause to pay attention as I had to keep up with the demands of work and life. I was once able to handle all of the work pressures and take up challenging projects but things had changed and accepting it, initially, felt like defeat in a way. I was nervous when I approached my husband to let him know I wanted to quit my job. When I said I wanted to talk to him in regards to my work, even without me saying it explicitly, my husband asked me to quit my job. He knew what I was going through and even though there were no real conversations on the amount of stress I endured in the past, he could sense it. When I heard what I wanted to hear, it gave me a great sense of assurance that I could move forward with this big decision. I quit my job on Mother's day and until this day, it was the best gift I ever gave myself. I was relieved to be able to make the decision, as my job stress was impacting my health in a great way and the only way to regain my vitality and bounce back to life meant taking the time and energy for self-care. The solitude meant more time for inner healing.

With my job and kids (for most part during the day) out of my life, I could feel the stress lifting off of my shoulders. There was an immense peace that I felt in my life after a long time of not feeling so. I was not able to pin point the real reason for the peace that I felt, neither was I in a mood to question it. All I wanted to do was to be engulfed in the peace and remain there.

> *Once the internal battle settles, we learn the art of letting go; acceptance becomes the next big step towards healing.*

I slept for more than 10-12 hours daily for the next few weeks. I think it was my body's way of surrendering and healing from within. I slowly began to accept and let go of some of my strong beliefs on perfectionism. When I reacted with anger or resentment towards something, I could recognize the symptoms my body was giving me. I used to have severe neck pain and felt the tightness in my shoulders and chest. There was heaviness weighing me down. I realized this was what I did to my body if I reacted the way I was not supposed to. With this realization my reaction times reduced drastically. I learnt to respond and speak things out clearly however uncomfortable it made me feel. When I did the right thing, I felt much more at peace with myself. What I once saw as a symptomatic body I later began to be more grateful for the signals it was giving me. When I used to be on Facebook with my phone and scroll down aimlessly, my wrist pains increased due to carpal tunnel, another symptom when you have thyroid issues. When I spent more time with unproductive tasks like watching TV for hours together, or spending a lot of time on technological gadgets like computers and phones or being on the phone for long hours right before bedtime, I used to feel completely drained. I listened to my body and I gathered my insights on my awareness.

When it came to diet, I realized having rice for lunch made me sleepy, sluggish and less productive - but rice was my go to comfort food and also when I felt more stressed that was the first food I always reached out for. I made a conscious decision to reduce it which did not help much so I replaced it with vegetables, beans and lentils for lunch. Paying attention to minute details like these throughout the day as I listened to my body started to become more intentional. I started to make conscious decisions throughout the day.

When I initially started to read about fatigue and energy during my early days of recovery it was the first drop in the ocean. I needed to gain the energy to do the things I used to love to do and to be totally there for my kids and my family. I used to say my energy has to be twice of where I currently am $Energy = MeenaChan^2$ and write down $E=MC^2$ back then.

- **Thoughts, words and actions - everything has energy.**

Out of the three choices for me, the easiest was to begin to work on my actions since the results were tangible. With my words I had to pay much more attention since it was not tangible right away, but my body displayed unpleasantness through pain and aches during times of anger or frustration. With the work stress relieved and kids being taken care of, I reduced my stress so that my anger and frustration levels also came down drastically. Afternoon naps rejuvenated me and I was in a better mental and emotional frame. I was more present when my kids and my husband came back home and could take care of them since I had the time to care for myself during the day. I lowered my expectations from others and from myself and began to express myself through writing them down.

Out of the three - thoughts, words and actions, being intentional with my thoughts was the most difficult for me. This illness made it easy for me even with my thoughts. I'm a thought lover and I love to just sit down and think for hours. It can be anything as simple as how can I improve on something to grand ideas. Hashimoto's made me brain-dead figuratively. I was so fatigued to even think any more that it greatly reduced my thought capacity. There was no thinking brain, just my soul speaking to me for the first time that I could actually hear it clearly. I felt the total silence, expansiveness and calmness deep down under all of the superficial chaos.

I felt Hashimoto's was not the end of the journey but the beginning to a new awakened life.

CHAPTER SEVEN
TRIP OVER TRANSITION

I kick started a rest, nourish and detox regime based on my ND's suggestion. I saw improvements with the quality of my sleep since letting go of the anxiety and stress of going to work the next day or caring for my kids for a few hours. Also the extra time I had during the day could now be spent on creating some fresh nourishing foods for myself. My body did not like the detox part initially as I experienced unpleasant reactions. I gave up sugar and felt physically run down and had spells of light headedness. In the morning, right after my kids and husband's send offs to school and work, I felt light headed and my body felt like it wanted to crash any moment. I was used to taking sugary foods for breakfast and with coffee, so as soon as I gave it up, my body went into shock and took time to get used to it. I also craved salty foods which is a common symptom when you have adrenal fatigue. During the initial stages of detox, I experienced severe headaches, abdominal cramps, more sluggishness and seemed more irritable too. Since I had experienced a whole range of symptoms and roller coaster of emotions earlier with the illness, symptoms arising due to the detox felt trivial. I took it one day at a time and if I happened to skip the sugar or rice for that day, then it was my personal victory and I had to repeat it the next day.

> *I did not think in terms of several days to weeks in advance which might have made me overwhelmed and cause me to stop in my tracks. I focused only on one day and for that moment.*

I was gradually making the changes, experimenting and at the same time observing my body's signals.

Experimentation + Observation = Wonders to your recovery

All throughout the journey I maintained transparency in communication with my ND taking note of what was working or not working with my body. **I kept a detailed food log taking note of what I ate from morning to evening. If a particular food made me feel unpleasant in any way, I had it down on the notes.** During my salt cravings, I used to head straight to a big pack of chips and would most times empty the entire pack in one sitting. Later I would regret the chip binge; I was bloated and stuffed up to my neck physically, mentally I felt sluggish and lacked clarity; emotionally I felt guilty. Consuming the entire pack only made me feel temporarily wonderful but then the misery set in later. I avoided the mindless craving for salty foods and substituted them with other nutritious snacks like nuts. Every time I overcame my little enemies, I felt victorious and I noticed the improvement in my mood as I had a sense of accomplishment. Remember, a medical practitioner can help in only the physical aspect of recovery and not be a guide through your holistic journey. I realized that health meant physical, mental, emotional and spiritual. The lessons learnt in one area can definitely be implemented in other areas too. Each stage I checked in, not only with my body but with my feelings too.

> *Feelings are true windows to your body. I used to have pause time set up on my phone calendar for four times during the day, twice before lunch and twice in the evening. I simply paused to observe how I was feeling.*

I began to realize something within me was gradually beginning to change. Self-awareness led to self-acceptance, I learned to respect my body and worked based on my strength, which I realized then was an intrapersonal skill, an ability to understand myself fully and work based on that. I was nowhere close to being where I wanted to be, but the belief was growing stronger that I could make it to where I wanted to be. With each opportunity I was trying to understand myself at a deeper level. The more things were becoming clearer the more questions it raised. I learnt to care for myself like you would protectively nurture a baby and went easy on myself during this journey. There were days I would experiment, observe and analyze and then days where I would do nothing but rest since that was what my body would have called out for that day. When I look back I realize that what I did then was immersing myself in self-compassion and trying not to be too hard or judgmental on myself. I knew deep within that I wanted to improve and get better in all aspects of life. I had to be clear with my destination which required me to chart out a route to take me there. When I rearranged my priorities, set my boundaries and was on a pursuit to improve my wellbeing, I felt Hashimoto's disorder was leading me to greater order. I had tripped onto defining my MOTTO. I realized I could transform the Hashimoto's and redefine it using my personal MOTTOs that I had discovered.

I strongly believe everything in life has a purpose and meaning, sometimes it's hard to realize this when we are amidst the struggle. I kept asking myself what can I learn from this? There must be a reason for this. If I had not thought beyond that stage my life would have been the same, working a full-time job, managing my family and going through life in a mundane way. There would have been no transformation emotionally, mentally or spiritually. Something has to breakdown to breakthrough. The health crisis I faced was a revelation in a sense. Some psychologists say that a psychological breakdown differs from a psychological rebirth, only by the end result. One leads to great health while the other leads to illness. Dr. Lisa Miller, Professor and Director of Clinical Psychology at Teacher's College, Columbia, states how women who have gone through suffering and pain and end up on spiritual paths, have nice thick cortexes. The back of their heads give out a certain wavelength of energy that is called 'alpha' that is also found on the back of the head of a meditating monk. Alpha has another name in Schumann's constant, it's the wavelength of the earth's crust. The spiritually engaged brain vibrates at the frequency of the earth's crust. Did I turn spiritual in one day? Not at all, but deep introspection sowed seeds for greater well-being.

Anthony Williams in his book, Thyroid Healing, talks about how the medical world believes that T3 and T4 are the only two main hormones the thyroid is responsible for and testing these would reveal the health of a patient's thyroid. He says, producing these hormones are one of the least important tasks of the thyroid as if it was, then they could be replaced by medication. However, the majority don't recover simply by medication, it happens to only to a small amount of people.

> *What truly makes the change are the positive lifestyle and the diet changes one makes.*

The way forward that exists is the strong belief that recovery is possible and that you have the choice to make yourself feel better. Contemplate on the two choices available, if you feel better how would your world change? And if you don't, what are some of the things you would lose? Is there value in staying stuck? If you chose not to believe in recovery, you might be caught in the endless loop of doctor visits, repeated tests to monitor your thyroid levels, consuming pills with no real improvement in the quality of your life and the amount of money, time and efforts that go in vain. Your entire life will be dulled down and lack the momentum and the joy as you're left at the mercy of the medication which ultimately, does nothing to your body. For me, my choice of belief was to recover completely so I could care for my family better and experience life to a much greater extent. Also I felt being healthy was my responsibility and one that should not be in the hands of others.

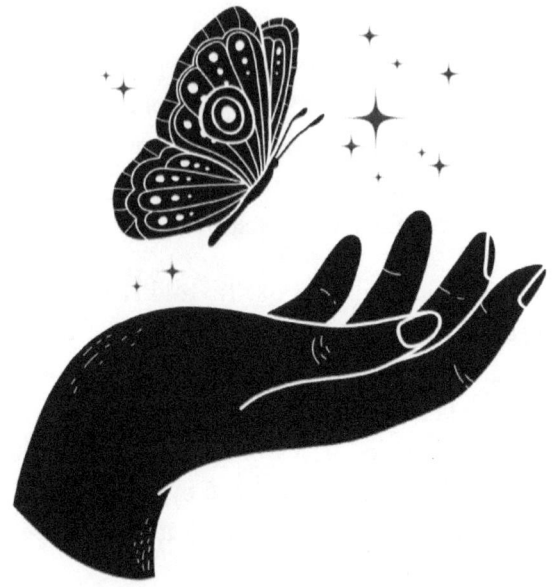

We all love to have great health and happiness and sometimes feel things are out of control and there is no way that we can make it happen. It once again comes back to thoughts, belief and trust.

▪ *Self-care begins with the right yes's and the right no's.*

Treat your body as a friend and that you are mutually helping each other out. The better we can take care of our body, the better our body can take us to our destination of where we want to be in our life. The journey ahead will take some time; it's taken a long time to get to this stage of struggle, ignoring the body signals all throughout, so it would take time to not only fully heal and recover, but in the process discover the transformation that accompanies the recovery. After much exploration and experimentation, I put together simple lifestyle changes that could help you reverse Hashimoto's or to go into remission.

The body and mind are wonderfully connected with each other; every thought can set off a series of reactions at the cellular level in our nervous system which has a great influence on all the cells in our body. Thoughts are the lighthouse to all the cells in our body guiding them to act and move accordingly. We need to ensure we have positive thoughts to help us to recover. Treating chronic illness holistically, as mind, body and spirit becomes imperative. Envision an equilateral triangle with the three aspects of mind, body and spirit. Even if one side of the triangle is lopsided or one aspect of your life is not in balance, then we cannot reach our true potential. Taking care of the mind is as important as taking care of the body or the spirit or vice versa.

Maslow said that if you plan on being anything less than you are capable of being, you will probably be unhappy all of the days of your life. We can take purposeful action even when we are feeling fatigued, anxious, depressed or fearful.

Get ready to commit yourself to live your life to the length, breadth and depths of it.

END OF PART TWO
CHECK-IN

1. Are you motivated to make lifestyle changes that will impact your overall health? Do pause and give this question consideration. This single decision could change your health and life's trajectory. (I'm sure the answer to this would be an astounding yes; otherwise you might have not gotten this far in this book).

_____
_____
_____
_____
_____
_____
_____

2. Are you aware of where your time goes? List 5 major activities that you did this week. How many of those were on self-care and how many were for others? Were those activities on your must do list or could have/ should have list? (Where your attention and time goes your energy goes there).

_____
_____
_____
_____
_____
_____
_____
_____

PART THREE
DISCOVERING MY MOTTO'S

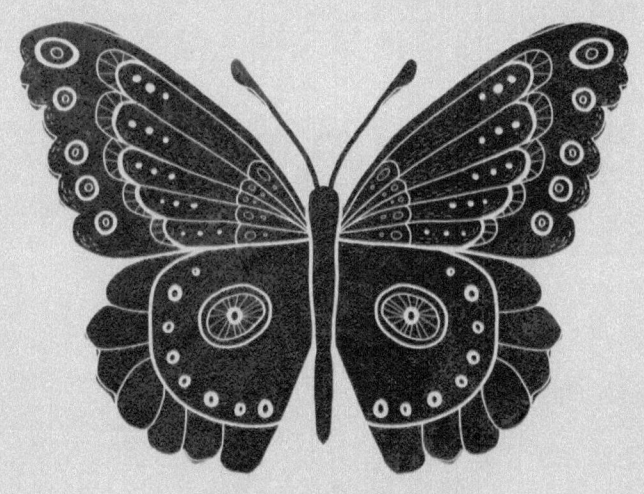

THE BODY MOTTO

What we do with our physical body such as exercise, sleep and diet, immensely impacts our mental state. There's a fascinating synergy between the mind, body and soul. On the overall wellbeing journey the easiest place to start would be the body. As easy as it may seem to start it does take dedication, commitment and patience. As mentioned earlier, I had a few basics in terms of diet and sleep set in motion working with my ND, however I did not have a clearly laid out strategy on what aspects of my body I needed to work on.

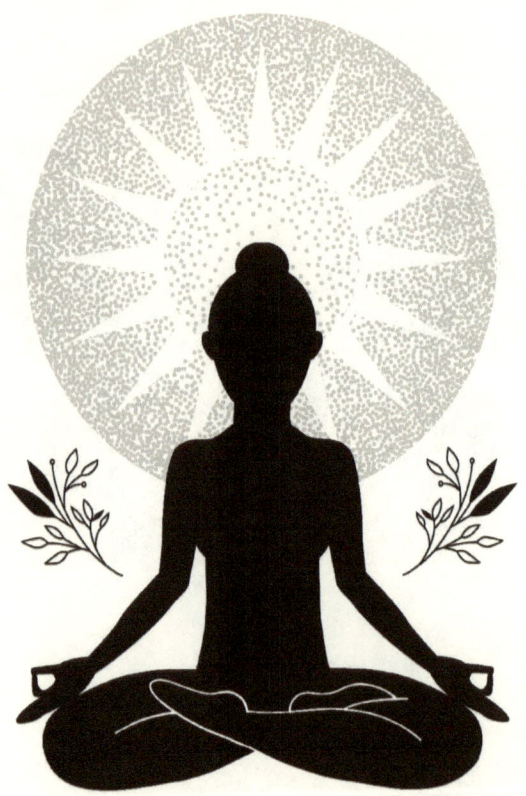

The yogic texts define the physical body and the vital force as sthula sharira, which means the 'gross body'. The mental body or the intellect as the sukshma sharia, which means the 'subtle' or the 'astral body' and finally the soul as karana sharira, or the 'causal body'. Plutarch, a Greek priest called them as the soma, psyche and nous. These are intricately linked and the way to reach your soul would be by working on the 'sheaths' or layers of the physical body and then to the mental body. Since the body is the most tangible form that can be perceived by our five senses, it was considered as a vehicle to reach the other levels such as the mind and the soul. The greater the functioning of the physical body, the greater are the chances to more fully engage with the mind and the soul. In the Body MOTTO we delve into four main aspects – The Moto MOTTO, The Yogic MOTTO, The Plateful MOTTO and the Marma MOTTO. These will help your body to function at its best and create a balance and harmony within your physical system. The greater the harmony, the greater the body is said to be at ease without 'dis-ease'.

CHAPTER EIGHT

THE MOTO MOTTO

'Moto' means movement or motion. The first place to start would be to move and keep the body physically active and engaged. Earlier in my journey, my movements were confined to the kitchen, refrigerator and pantry, to the couch. I used to sit for 8-10 long hours working on my laptop, then when kids came along I used to sit down to feed them for 30 minutes for each feed and 8-10 times per day, which equaled to 4 hours and more. Only the places where I sat down changed, but physically there was no change in my fitness levels. My number one reason I always had was "I have no time." Before kids, my fingers had good exercise moving up, down, right and left on the television remote for hours on the weekends. Back then I did not have the desire or the need to exercise. The desire to get healthy, recover and heal was so strong later on that I began to find the time and the motivation to exercise. **The Centers for Disease and Control suggests that people get at least 150 minutes of moderate activity each week (30 minutes a day) coupled with two or more days of muscle-strengthening activity.**

WALKING

I started with walking 30 minutes each day and later increased it to an hour each day. Initially, even just a few minutes into walking I would feel breathless and light headed. I took it slow; my pace was initially slower too and I gradually increased it. I got myself a basic Fitbit tracker that would track the number of steps and calories. My goal was only to get more active and energetic and was not to lose weight. I used to be lean before I had kids and later I had lost all the post pregnancy weight too (thanks to hyperthyroidism that I had for a few months!) The Fitbit tracker really kept me motivated to do more and I enjoyed seeing the number of steps increasing when I walked. My everyday to-do list had walking right at the top so I made it a conscious decision to complete it every day. The recommended daily goal is 10,000 steps. The Japanese first popularized the manpo-kei which means a 10,000 steps meter, which was adopted by other pedometers too. I was able to do 100 steps per minute which meant I needed to do 60 minutes to complete 6000 steps. My average steps spent doing chores and other activities came to 3000-4000 steps; the days it was lower it meant I had to walk further.

BENEFITS OF WALKING

> *Research has shown that walking 10,000 steps per day can lead to a decrease in chronic illnesses like diabetes and heart diseases.*

In one study it was found that postal workers in Glasgow, Scotland, who walked 15,000 steps a day, had fewer risk factors for heart disease than colleagues who sat throughout the day[1].

• Walking improves fitness, reduces body fat and body weight, improves mood and alleviates depression and fatigue, improves endurance, posture and circulation.

• Walking is a zero investment activity and a perfect beginner exercise. You don't have to buy those fancy workout clothes, or spend a lot, but can experience the benefits of all those workouts and more with this simple exercise that you can fit into a daily routine.

• Walking has several mental and emotional benefits as well. One Stanford University study found that walking increased creative output by an average of 60 percent. Researchers labeled this type of creativity "divergent thinking," which they define as a thought process used to generate creative ideas by exploring many possible solutions[2]. According to the study, "walking opens up the free flow of ideas, and it is a simple and robust solution to the goals of increasing creativity and increasing physical activity." Your creativity peaks and it allows your mind to be more favorable for innovative ideas.

- *Psychologists found that 10 minutes of walking everyday may be just as good as a 45 minutes workout to relieving symptoms of anxiety.*

During my walks I always tried to accomplish tasks like checking emails, or having a phone conversation with my parents, or one of my favorite activities was to watch or listen to informational trainings, interviews or talks in the area of my interest and take notes on my phone. I would also review my goals and make notes on improvements. I felt walking helped me with problem solving or coming up with fresh ideas for improvements more than any other activity. When I had something that required thinking time, or a task that I could do whilst on the go, I would make a note of it on my phone and take it up during my daily walk. I made good use of that time and I looked forward to it. Most days I was so engrossed in learning on the move that up to an hour and half would have gone by without me realizing it. Some days having a solid hour dedicated to walking was not possible, so I used to split it up with 20 minutes in the morning, 20 minutes after lunch and 20 minutes after dinner. This kept it more achievable and also walking after a meal improved my digestion to a great extent too. Walking post lunch also helped with the sluggishness and brain fog I felt sometimes after I had consumed a high carb meal and I instantly noticed the attentiveness and surge of energy by doing so. Or the alternative approach would be to complete more steps during the start of the day so you have less to catch up on later. Walking is a lower impact exercise that can be done for longer periods of time. Personally, if there's just one exercise that I could choose to do in a day for 15-20 minutes then it would be to walk.

HIGH-INTENSITY WORKOUTS

High-intensity workouts alternate between intense bursts of activity and fixed periods of less-intense activity or even complete rest. It is a cardio vascular exercise strategy. For example, a good starter workout is running as fast as you can for 1 minute and then walking for 2 minutes. People with Hashimoto's or underactive thyroid need to avoid high-intensity activities at the beginning. Choose a low impact activity to start with and then let your body gradually ease into the exercise rhythm. You may later pick activities that suit your body and its needs. Regular exercise will help to manage your symptoms better. Before I joined a gym, one of my primary concerns was my fatigue and if I might be able to work out or if those activities might do me more harm? I realized that with regular exercise I felt a lot better physically, mentally and emotionally. I felt more energized and could carry out the daily activities with more ease and zest. I had enough energy day-to-day and more energy to run around and play with my kids, take them out to different places and enjoy spending bountiful time in taking care of them. I was mentally prepared and took a firm decision before joining a gym which helped me to stay committed. For me personally, once I take the time and energy to think through things I am ready to commit to it and do not allow it to fizzle out; such as not going to the gym, since I had a strong why behind it that kept me motivated. I joined one of the premier gyms in the city, so it was a big financial decision as well. I used to joke that my inspiration was my husband's perspiration, but I felt I would rather invest in my fitness and health than paying up for doctor visits. The gym had the finest of trainers and instructors.

I did an hour of yoga, 45 minutes of strength or cardio and 30 minutes of walking on the treadmill every day. I later added swimming and my walking turned into jogging and then running. Each day I tried out different classes to know which one suited me best and also depending on the way that I felt that day. One day I was prepared to go into my restorative yoga class but it got cancelled unexpectedly and the only other class that day during that time, was a high intensity dancercise. I did not know what to expect and went into the class. I anticipated a relaxing class that day but ended up with an action packed class and I loved it. Dancercise was fast paced and every time I tried to co-ordinate the leg movements, my hands were off, and vice versa which made me focus all of my attention on my trainer and I never realized how quick the time went by. Also with that one class, my regular chores and other activities, I was able to complete 10,000 steps which meant I did not need to do any extra walking that day! Once a week gave myself a break from walking and chose a high intensity class which worked out great for my energy levels too.

I gradually worked towards increasing the intensity of my work outs. That year I had a goal of getting out of my comfort zone and I really stretched myself. I asked myself what was my number one fear and I would take up that activity to challenge it so that my confidence level increased. For me it was swimming, I used to panic just at the thought of getting into the water. I joined an adult's swim lesson, so I did not have to dread the fact that young swimmers would get to watch me. My first day, waddling through the water made me feel so unsteady. For months I struggled to let go of the pool wall which made me feel safe. I used to prepare my mind and give myself a pep talk each time I went into the pool but as soon as I was chest deep in the water, fear would take over and I panicked. I kept at it, watched videos, took extra swim lessons and practiced by myself three times a week. I'm still not there yet, but this gave me great confidence in knowing that I worked on my number one fear and I realized that I did have good self-regulation and discipline for which I patted myself on my back.

Remember that with hypothyroidism you might have to work harder towards losing weight than someone without thyroid disease, but the mental and emotional benefits make it worth the effort to exercise by far.

Here's a list of beginner exercises you could consider:
- Walking
- Bike riding or indoor cycling
- Elliptical training
- Stair climbing
- Yoga
- Tai Chi
- Hiking on easy terrain
- Dancing
- Swimming
- Strength training
- Barre
- Pilates
- Any sports

Here's a list of more advanced exercises you could consider if you feel you're ready for it:
- High intensity interval training (HIIT)
- Aerobics
- Zumba

- Running / Marathons
- Hot Yoga
- All activities listed in the beginner exercises but with more intensity

Below is my sample schedule that I follow.

SAMPLE SCHEDULE

MON	TUE	WED	THU	FRI	SAT	SUN
Vinyasa Yoga	Muscle	High-intensity interval training	Barre			
At home: meditation and walking 10,000 steps each				At home: meditation, extensive yoga and walking 10,000 steps each day		

Choose activities that work for you and based on your level of interest.

If you're a morning person you could try to get the activities accomplished in the morning so it gives you a burst of energy throughout the day, if you are a night owl, then you can focus on the evenings since it would give you more energy towards the end of your day. For me personally, a three-day rest and restore regime suited me well with my activities done at home and 4 times a week I enjoyed my work outs at the gym. A few things, such as having the best workout clothes that fit you perfectly, including the right undergarments, can make a world of difference. When I had to do push-ups which were hard for me, instead of counting from one to twenty, I used to count from twenty to one, in reverse. I felt it gave me a push to reach one, instead of the pull and struggle to reach twenty. I'm not sure how that really works, but it's my personal hack that always did the trick. I had the base number twenty already set firmly in my mind and all I had to do was to reach one which felt more achievable. The days when you don't feel like heading to the gym, the trick is to get dressed quickly and head out of the door leaving you with no room to think and give into that feeling. The moment you hit the class, the feeling of not wanting to go subsides and you come out of the class feeling much stronger than ever since you have learnt the art of self-empowerment!

Here's how I felt when I initially started to work out, which could provide you with some inspiration. My goal was not to lose weight since I was on the lean side, but I did end up losing weight. If your goal is to lose weight, then this should make you more encouraged! If you're the type who would aspire to check their biceps in the mirror each week, the below information should give you a realistic deadline too. For the first 12 weeks just keep at it and eventually you will begin to notice the results.

Be result-driven but action oriented and focus on the process.

I used to take it one day at a time and during the class my focus was on the trainer and making sure I did as much as I could of what was taught and that simply kept me going. There was no right or wrong way, I've had my fair share of stumbles and laughed about it. As a beginner, I've had the wobbly legs after workouts and had to hold onto the staircase railing to walk downstairs. I had days where I felt I progressed much quicker and took two steps forward only to realize I had to take four steps backward and slow down. I had a time when I felt sick after over exhaustion and my workouts came to a grinding halt. At that time coming to a halt was not the struggle, but getting started again was the hard part. What I had gained after months of perseverance was lost within two weeks and I felt that was unfair.

THE PROGRESS CHART

• **First 4 weeks:** Felt extremely tired and body soreness for three days. My sleep improved

• **After 4 weeks:** Felt lighter

• **After 6 weeks:** Endurance, stamina, exhaustion levels, breathlessness improved

• **After 8 weeks:** Felt good mood wise, felt more positive, legs felt tighter/stronger, my abs felt a little toned

• **After 10 weeks:** Lost 3 pounds, slept better, felt more productive and was able to finish up my work faster, worked from 5.15am till 9.30pm with no sleep, stopped my naps, able to lift weights better.

> *Working on the physical fitness has tremendous impact on your mental health. It expands your self-confidence and your sense of self-definition to great heights. You learn a great deal about what your body can and cannot do which is no longer a limitation since you gain the belief that you can defy those limits.*

As the definition of yourself keeps expanding, it spills out to other aspects of your life too. I felt energized, my creative juices began to flow, ideas began to evolve and my productivity peaked. I completed all of the tasks I had on my to-do list for that day and began to take up tasks from the next day too!

What's your MOTTO?

CHECK IN

1. Do you currently have a fitness routine in place?
_____

2. Do you meet the recommended 30 minutes of exercise per day?
_____

3. If not, is there any activity that you are currently interested in?
(Example: dancing or a sport that you always wanted to try?)
_____

4. What's the number one thing that is stopping you from getting started on your fitness journey?
_____

5. What's one thing you would like to overcome with your health?
(Example: overcome fatigue, lose weight, overcome muscle weakness)
_____

6. What's one step, you can take towards getting started on your fitness journey?
_____

7. Imagine how you would like to feel physically?
(Example: Fit, toned, healthy, improve your stamina, endurance, filled with vitality, gain muscle strength)
_____

SUMMARY

- The body is the most tangible form that can be perceived by our five senses, it is considered as a vehicle that helps us reach our mind and the soul.

- 'Moto' means movement or motion. The first place to start would be to move and keep your body physically active and engaged.

- The Centers for Disease and Control suggests that people get at least 150 minutes of moderate activity each week (30 minutes a day) coupled with two or more days of muscle-strengthening activity.

WALKING

- Research has shown that with adequate other healthy habits, walking 10,000 steps per day can lead to a decrease in chronic illnesses like diabetes and heart diseases.

- Walking is the perfect beginner workout that improves fitness, reduces body fat and body weight, improves mood and alleviates depression and fatigue, improves endurance, posture and circulation.

- Walking is a zero investment activity and a perfect beginner exercise.

- Think of activities that engage you during your walks so you get to enjoy your walks more and prefer not to skip it.

- Walking can help to get your creative juices flowing called the 'divergent thinking'.

- Psychologists found that 10 minutes of walking everyday maybe just as good as 45 minutes workout to relieving symptoms of anxiety.

HIGH-INTENSITY WORKOUTS

- High intensity workouts is a cardio vascular strategy that alternates between intense bursts of activity and fixed periods of less-intense activity.

- You may choose a low impact activity to start with and then let your body gradually ease into the exercise rhythm.

- With regular exercise you will feel a lot better physically, mentally and emotionally. It expands your self-confidence and your sense of self-definition to great heights.

CHAPTER NINE
THE YOGIC MOTTO

If there's a perfect secret sauce to nurture your body, mind and soul at the same time then it would be yoga. The secret ingredient in the sauce is the breath, which unites all three aspects. Through breath one has direct access to controlling the prana or the life force. If any of the pretzel poses or upside down contractions look daunting to you, then you can be assured that yoga is simply not being like Elasti-girl that you see in the animation movie The Incredibles. Elasti-girl is a dexterous superheroine who can stretch any part of her body and mold it into any shape or size. Yoga includes a series of body postures and moving to the rhythms of in and out breath combined with mindfulness that can help with strengthening the mind body connection. It is derived from the Sanskrit word 'yuji' meaning yoke or union, an ancient practice that brings union of the mind and body.

I was introduced to yoga when I was 11 years old; I began a class but did not sustain it since I lacked the interest. Then at 16, I attended a class and kept at it much longer than the first time. It was a group class where we were taught surya namaskars or sun salutations which are a series of yoga poses that are done as 12 sets, and each set has 12 asanas each side, which means you would end up doing 288 poses! I felt it was too intense and required too much time commitment to perfect the poses and dropped out of the class. During my early 20s, I had worked my way to burnout during my career and got introduced to yoga once again. I had experienced severe neck pain and nothing could help alleviate the pain. I had tried physiotherapy, x-rays and medications. Yoga was the only modality that helped at that time. I went to a well-known yoga therapy school that teaches students poses specifically targeted to their illness. I then practiced yoga for next 10 years, there were months I used to be super dedicated and months where I totally skipped it. During pregnancy and after my kids were born the routine was out of place. If I had to reduce my anxiety and calm down physically, mentally and emotionally, I intuitively knew the answer was to get back to yoga. I knew that the benefits I felt when I initially began to work on it were substantial, no matter what happened in the outside world, I could choose to remain calm within by consistent practice.

When I had joined the gym, they had several yoga classes taught by excellent teachers. The group yoga classes were welcoming, people came from different backgrounds, some have worked out intensely and others have never worked out before. I learnt to understand my body's limits and to push through and find comfort in my discomfort so that my body learnt to adjust and expand to meet the new goals. Yoga is perfect for pre body workout as you get to stretch your muscles and this helps prevent soreness and injury during other workouts. You can even do a quick stretch anytime during the day to take a break from long hours of work, especially if you have a desk based sedentary job.

BENEFITS OF YOGA

- Can reduce stress, multiple studies have shown that it can reduce the secretion of cortisol - the primary stress hormone.

- Helps relieve anxiety, bringing the awareness to present moment can help calm down the parasympathetic nervous system.

- Can help reduce inflammation, consistent practice has shown to help increase the immunity and bring down the inflammatory markers in the body.

- Helps improve overall blood circulation and thereby can help improve heart health.

- Helps lower the levels of depression, since a decrease in the cortisol levels also influences the levels of serotonin, the neurotransmitter associated with depression.

- Helps reduce chronic pain with symptoms like carpal tunnel and osteoarthritis and it's a low impact exercise.

- Enhances sleep quality because of its effect on melatonin, a hormone that regulates sleep.

Here are some tips for beginners, if you would like to consider Yoga in your fitness regime.

- Start slowly and ease into it. There are some basic stretches and warm ups that you could immensely benefit from

- Find a teacher who can guide you through the process. If you are new to it, then the best place to start might be at a group yoga class offered at the gym or even an exclusive yoga studio

- If cost is a concern, then opt for a gym rather than the studios. You could even do a trial class at the gym or at the yoga studio to see how you like it. The places that offer yoga also provide the mats and equipment needed, however if you wish, you may take your own yoga mat for the classes too.

- Be consistent and keep at it since you will see the benefits gradually, however, these are long term. Meaning that once you set the right foundation, the benefits can last for a long time.

- Do not compare yourself with the pros and yoga is not merely doing some acrobatic poses and complex twists. Yoga is about creating an internal union and this can be done without those twists too.

• Hydrate yourself well prior to and post class, so it can help flush out the toxins from the body.

HASHIMOTO'S TARGETED YOGA POSES

I attended different yoga classes that were offered at the gym—Vinyasa, Restorative, Yin Yang, Yoga flow, Hatha, Yoga Nidra and Hot yoga. There are many more which can be an overwhelming choice for beginners. By attending a variety of classes, I learnt what personally worked for me and made me feel good from within. The longer you practice the more you will realize what suits your body and later you get to intuitively go with the flow of the poses. Each body type is unique, what may suit one may not be the best solution for another. Think of an all you can eat menu being served, you choose what you like and leave out the rest. Similarly, you may adopt practices that work for your body and omit the rest. Experiment and see what works for your body under the guidance of a good yoga teacher. Go back to your symptoms and consider yoga as your therapy, specifically addressing that particular area. I had to work on my fatigue, overall stress, digestion, body pains and the thyroid of course. Yoga really helped me overcome my stress and anxiety in a big way, leaving me energized and rejuvenated after a session.

> *Since a lot of emotional tensions are stored in the body, yoga can help open up those areas to enable you to release those emotions that are holding you back.*

Below are some of the yoga poses I consistently practice every single day. There are some more that I do, but these 11 poses are the non-negotiables in my practice and I never skip on these.

***I'm not a certified yoga teacher, so these poses are to be attempted under the guidance of a yoga teacher. Also if you are pregnant, or have other chronic conditions, you need to exercise caution as these may not be suitable for you.

1. CHILD'S POSE or BALASANA

This is a beginner pose that stretches the muscles of the lower back and inner thighs. It promotes stress relief, flexibility and helps with circulation to the muscles, back and hips.

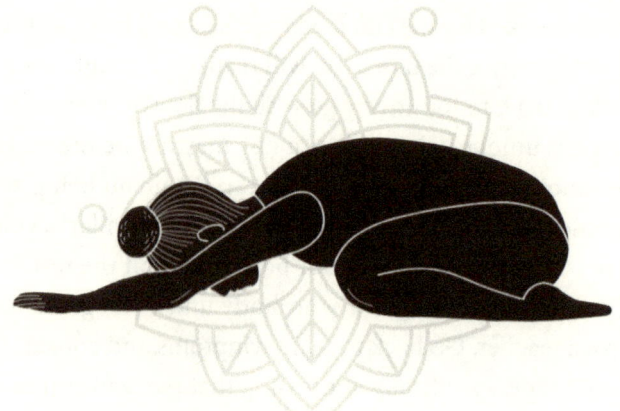

This is a hip opener pose, the emotional purpose behind this pose is to have more flexibility in life. You will slowly begin to see the connection with thyroid and how some of these poses can help open up the tightness in the body and the emotional inflexibilities we hold onto in our lives. Rigidness and control affects the hips, which is the root area where the spine rests. This pose is deeply relaxing and can be done in between the poses. Taking time to rest in your practice may actually help you to cultivate the ability to take time out in your everyday life. You may find that you are better able to stop and re-charge your batteries.

2. CAT AND COW POSE or MARJARYASANA AND BITILASANA

Moving to the rhythmic breath movements the asana or the pose flows from cow tilt to cat stretch. This is a powerful pose for the mind, increases co-ordination and invigorates the prana - the life force within the body.

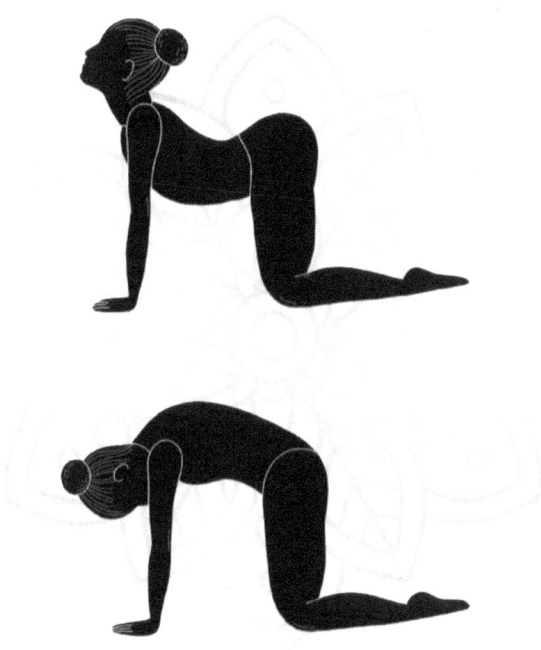

It increases the emotional balance and mind stability. The pose has tremendous benefits – it helps relieve menstrual cramps, lower back pain, sciatica, toning the gastrointestinal track and the female reproductive system. This activates the Swadisthana Chakra, the second chakra, which can help overcome deep emotional turmoil and depression. It also enhances creativity and the ability to focus and learn, which helps to combat the brain fog faced during Hashimoto's.

3. CAMEL POSE or USTRASANA

The Camel pose can be alternated with the child's pose. Where the child's pose is a forward bend, this one is a backward bend. You could take this up based on your comfort level and it may not be easy for a beginner.

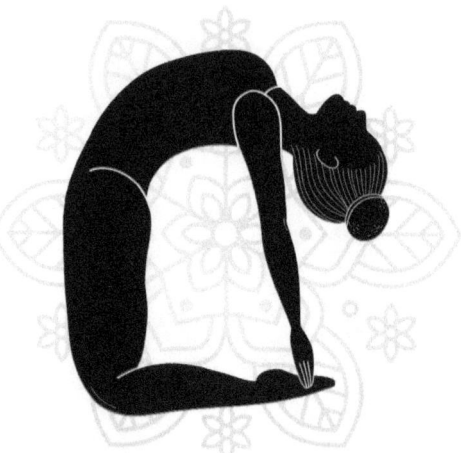

Also it's important to learn the right way to reach this pose. This helps improve spinal flexibility, strengthening the back muscles and also with improving the posture. With months of breastfeeding or working on the computer, the posture is compromised and this was one of the poses that really helped me with the posture. It also opens up the chest and lungs and will help increase the breathing capacity, improves digestion and stimulates the thyroid. It is said to tone the thighs, rejuvenate the energy levels and lower blood pressure. When you open up to this pose, mentally you open up as well, since this links to your heart chakra called the Anahata, the energy center for love, caring and compassion and you tend to look up to the possibilities.

4. COBRA POSE or BHUJANGASANA

This can be done based on your comfort level and there are

mini cobra poses too. Where the stretch is not too intense and you get to stretch only from the chest up and not all the way up like in the diagram.

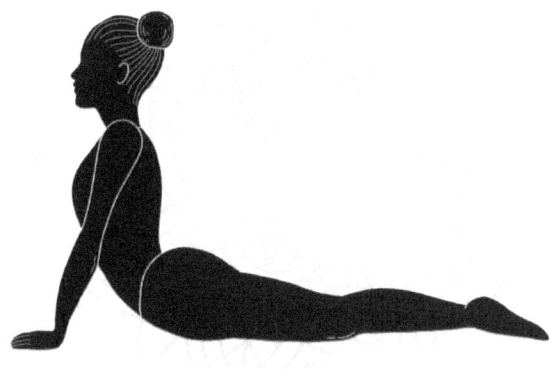

During this pose, there is a lot of compressing and stretching which helps in regulating the thyroid glands. This pose helps to strengthen your spine and shoulders, helps relieve stress and fatigue, soothes the sciatica, firms your buttocks, improves digestion and reduces back and neck pain. Begin slowly with a mild stretch and you may work your way up to the big stretch. Also if you are a runner this pose could help ease out the tighter muscles in front of your hips.

5. DOWNWARD FACING DOG POSE or ADHO MUKHA SVANASANA

This is one of my personal favorites and has so many benefits. With this pose I'm able to identify which part of my body is tight, sore or flexible. This can work out any kink in the body so it's crucial to learn the right way of doing this so that you can reap all of the benefits this pose provides. It lengthens, strengthens and energizes every muscle in your body and encourages blood flow to the brain. As you let your neck hang long, it releases tension from the back of your neck. This pose can recharge your batteries and are good for the wrists and can prevent carpal tunnel syndrome.

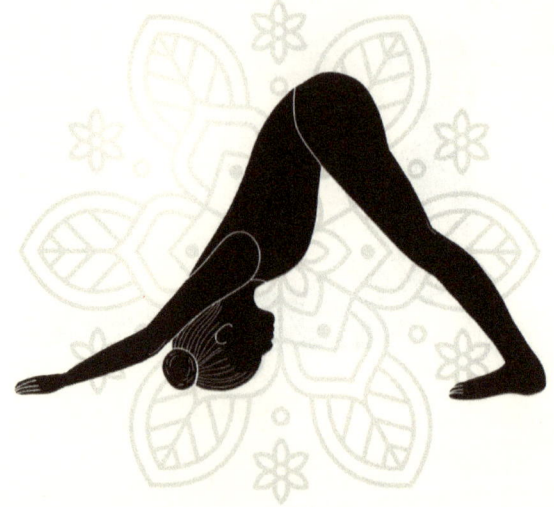

You may "walk your dog" where you tend to lift your heels up and down and also sway your hips side to side wagging your dog's tail.

6. GARLAND POSE *or* MALASANA

This pose helps to strengthen the ankles, lower hamstrings, groins, calf muscles, core and back.

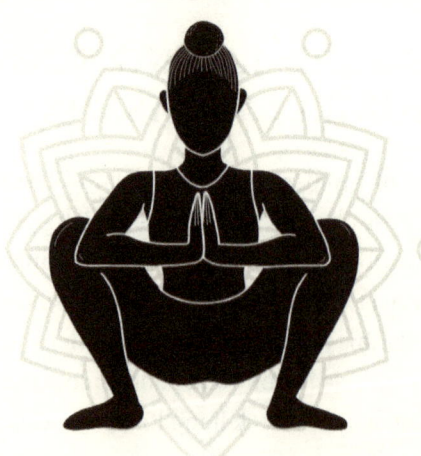

It has many physical, mental and spiritual benefits and calms the mind, body and spirit. Constant sitting can impair our lumbar (the lower region of our spine). This pose helps ease the hips open and increases the mobility of hips and legs. Since the body is closer to the earth, this activates the first chakra, muladhara, associated with safety and trust and has a powerful grounding quality. This pose is also called a relieving pose and can help with elimination, digestion and emotionally relieving negative thoughts.

7. MOUNTAIN POSE or TADASANA

This is a fundamental asana for all levels of yoga and has several physical, mental and spiritual benefits. I love to stand with my palms facing forward, to help open the heart and send energy down the arms to the ground.

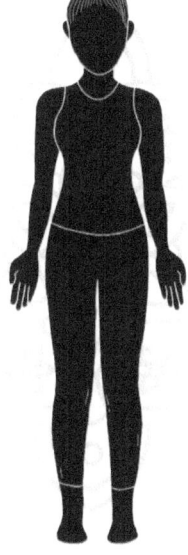

This pose helps strengthen the thighs, knees and ankles. Standing in stillness cultivates space for the body to pause and rest for digestion and circulation. It activates the inner fire and helps reduce depression. Mentally, it promotes an increased awareness of the mind and body and offers grounding effects. The spiritual benefits are that it activates the prana, or the life force within the body. This pose reinforces the aspect of mindfulness.

8. SHOULDER STAND POSE or SARVANGASANA

This helps in stimulating the thyroid glands and controls thyroxin. The blood flows from the legs to the head region due to the inverted pose which helps in mitigating thyroid. It helps improve digestion and elimination.

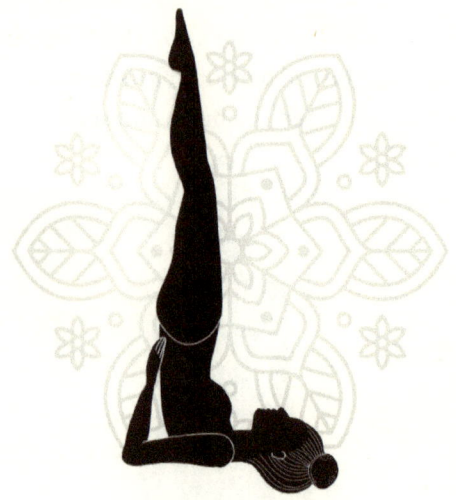

There's less strain on the heart since the heart does not have to work as hard to pump blood to various parts of the body. The lymphatic system is stimulated and it helps to boost your immune system. It helps to relieve nasal congestion, headaches and insomnia too. During menstruation this pose is not recommended.

9. PLOUGH POSE or HALASANA

This pose assists in balancing the glandular secretions, adrenaline and thyroxin, while also improving the elimination of toxins in the digestive and urinary tracts. Those with a tendency toward high blood pressure may find relief from hypertension in the pose. In the inverted position of Plough Pose, the brain is flushed with blood, promoting mental clarity and increased vitality. The pose resembles the Indian plough, hence it is called Halasana.

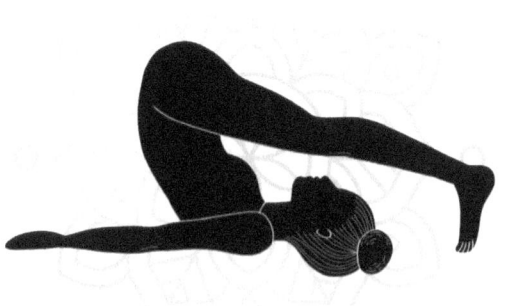

This has a calming, restorative effect on the sympathetic nervous system.

10. FISH POSE or MATSYASANA

This pose takes the form of a fish and therefore, it is called the Matsyasana.

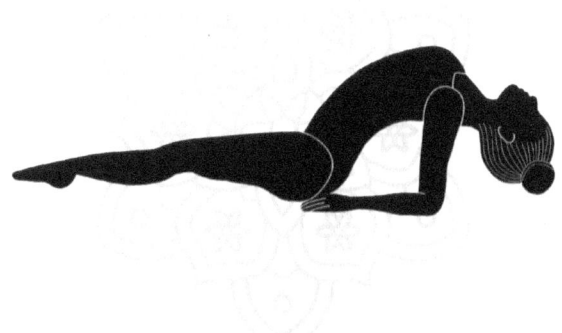

It stretches your neck hence stimulating the thyroid glands. This asana provides gentle healing suited to the needs of thyroid patients, lowers stress levels and reduces the stiffness of muscles and joints. It helps in relaxing the body and preventing mood swings and depression which thyroid might cause.

11. BRIDGE POSE or SETHUBANDHASANA

If you are able to perform the bridge pose successfully, it allows you to stretch your neck to quite an extent and activate the thyroid glands. It helps in calming the brain, reducing anxiety and improving the digestive system.

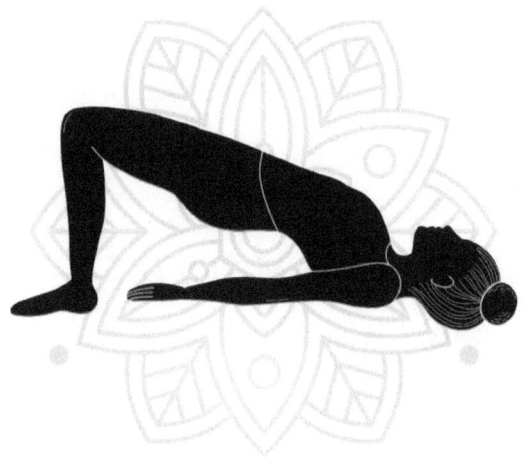

There is also the king of all poses, the Headstand pose or Sirshana. It is one of the finest yoga postures as it is turns your body upside down and rests the entire body on your head - it helps in managing the thyroid. It aids in balancing the metabolic functions and brings wakefulness and alertness to the body. Although this is something personally I have never attempted.

The above postures can be done at varying degrees of mindfulness and breath rhythm making it an exhilarating experience.

If yoga is not your kind of exercise, then you could try other exercises like Qi gong, Tai chi, Pilates or Barre, since any form of exercise is showing love to your body. The Yogic MOTTO and the Zen MOTTO (see under the Mind MOTTO section) go hand in hand, where you will learn how to exercise greater mind control.

If physical fitness through exercise is the first step towards self-definition, self-empowerment and self-respect, yoga is the first step towards building a connection with your mind and body and defining your self-discipline.

The learnings from yoga can be used anywhere in your life's journey throughout and you will see how these have a positive influence on the other aspects of your life since you are building the foundation to a great character.

What's your MOTTO?

CHECK-IN

1. Do you currently have Yoga, Qi Gong or Tai Chi as part of your routine?
_____
_____

2. Do you have an instructor to guide you? If not, look up studios or gyms that offer these and check out a trial class.
_____
_____

3. Identify your top 3 health concerns so you can customize your yoga poses to target those areas of concern in your body.
_____
_____

4. Check in with your body to see how you feel after a yoga session.
_____
_____

5. What are your top concerns that are currently stopping you from getting started with a fitness regime?
_____
_____

6. What are some of your solutions to work around above concerns?
_____
_____

SUMMARY

- Yoga means 'union', union or connection with your body and mind.

- Yoga can help reduce stress, inflammation, anxiety, chronic pains and helps improve the blood circulation and the quality of your sleep.

- Since a lot of emotional tensions are stored in the body, yoga can help open up those areas to enable you to release those emotions that are holding you back.

- If yoga is not your kind of exercise, then you could try other exercises like Qi gong, Tai chi, Pilates or Barre, since any form of exercise is showing love to your body.

- If physical fitness through exercise is the first step towards self-definition, self-empowerment and self-respect, yoga is the first step towards building a connection with your mind and body and defining your self-discipline.

CHAPTER TEN
THE PLATEFUL MOTTO

Ayurveda is one of the holistic healing systems which was developed 3,000 years ago in India, it states that one of the most important things we can do for our health is to eat wisely every day. 'Food is medicine' when consumed properly - you are what you eat. This means, all I was back then was a bag of potato chips, as that is what I consumed the most. Take this simple test and answer this question. What are you now? What does your daily diet look like? What you consume for the most part during the day is what you are going to be.

During my school and college days I was skinny. It took dedicated effort from one of my best friends, who is now a renowned chef, to help me gain a few pounds after numerous brownies, puddings and late night milk shakes during night overs that we shared. She loved to cook, I loved to eat and we were perfect for each other. For four years, being pregnant, feeding and raising two kids back to back, my body was trained to keep eating. Later when diagnosed with Hashimoto's, I had several digestive issues, abdominal cramps, headaches, bloating and constipation. Everything I ate caused me an issue of some sort. I once broke out into severe hives all over my body and did not know what the cause was. My body reacted to foods I was consuming then. Not only that, it was hard to shake off the weight I had gained during pregnancy due to hypothyroidism. Later, I lost a lot of weight and was back to my original weight with hyperthyroidism. Food and diet has always been an area of struggle for me. Not because I ate a lot, but due to the unhealthy food types I chose, and the consciousness I lacked about being intentional in what I consumed. I began to make a food log and track what I was eating during the day and how I felt eating those foods. Most times I knew that I may feel bad after eating a certain food, however, due to lack of choices I gave myself, I would end up eating the same things and feel miserable later on.

My ND suggested that I needed to fix the root cause of this illness and I had to take a good hard look at what I ate. I had a food allergy test done to identify if there were any foods that caused an allergic reaction to my body. It may also be used to find out whether you have a true allergy or instead, a sensitivity to a food. Food sensitivity, also called food intolerance, is often confused with a food allergy. The two conditions can have similar symptoms, but complications can be very different. A food allergy is an immune system reaction that can affect organs throughout the body. It can cause dangerous health conditions. Food sensitivity is usually much less serious. If you have food sensitivity, your body can't properly digest a certain food, or a food bothers your digestive system. Symptoms of food sensitivity are mostly limited to digestive problems such as abdominal pain, nausea, gas, and diarrhea.

When I took the food allergy test it was a real eye opener and downright depressing, because every single food I was eating until that point showed up in the food intolerance chart! When you have foods that you're sensitive or intolerant to, you need to avoid those foods for a certain period of time until your system heals. I was depressed because I did not know how to go about identifying new foods to eat. I'm also a choosy eater and I had never experimented much with different foods. The changes in my diet were a challenge to me physically, mentally and emotionally. When I was hungry I could not just grab any snack and eat it, I had to be conscious of what I was consuming. I had to plan in advance and make my lunch, dinner, breakfast and snacks which meant time management and a lifestyle change. I could not imagine how the simple diet changes could rock my entire life. I had to give up dairy, gluten, sugar, corn, soy, coconut, rice, grains, lentils, beans, night shade vegetables and all nuts. I was a vegetarian all throughout my growing up years so I did not have much choice. I wondered what was left to eat. I frantically went over the allergy test report to see what happened to coffee and chocolates. Thankfully, those came clear which meant I could have those. Before I started my elimination diet, I gave myself a week to prepare for the new diet changes. I took a day to mourn, three days to plan what to eat, two days to shop and a day to mentally get ready before I took the plunge. The journey through the diet changes were not easy at all, nevertheless it was totally worth the effort. If you are like me, and unsure of where to start, below are some tips on how I got started with the changes.

THE DIET ROADMAP

Step 1: Begin with a food log

Track what you eat from morning to night and write it down. There are several free food tracking apps too, however I personally love a pen and paper because it forces you to focus on what you write and it literally screams back at you! Emotionally, you may feel resistance to write it down, feel lazy to track it every day, feel guilty looking at what you ate and even angry, because what's the whole idea of this exercise. The first step is awareness. There are no judgements being made at this stage. You simply write what you eat. Continue to do this for two weeks.

SAMPLE FOOD LOG

BREAKFAST	coffee, donuts
IN BETWEEN	coffee, chips, nuts
LUNCH	burger and fries
SNACK	coffee, pretzels, brownies
IN BETWEEN	nuts
DINNER	chicken, beans, chocolate pudding
LATE NIGHT	popcorn, wine

Step 2: Circle the culprits

Even before my food allergy test I knew some of the foods that clearly I had to avoid. I wanted to escape the whole exercise of taking a good hard look at my diet since I was reluctant to change. There were a few that I did not expect, but for the most part, if we are honest and true to ourselves we know the culprits. From your food log, circle the ones you wish to avoid. Again, no judgements, do not plan ahead and wonder how you can live without those foods. *The second step is focus.* We are simply narrowing down and bringing our awareness to certain foods.

SAMPLE FOOD LOG

BREAKFAST	coffee, *donuts*
IN BETWEEN	*coffee, chips, nuts*
LUNCH	*burger and fries*
SNACK	coffee, pretzels, *brownies*
IN BETWEEN	nuts
DINNER	chicken, beans, chocolate pudding
LATE NIGHT	*popcorn, wine*

Step 3: Plan your replacements

Something has to be introduced for the existing food item to go out. I used to crave salty crunchy foods so I would always reach out for the bag of potato chips. If I had to choose a healthier alternative that had a similar texture and was a bit salty, I went for nuts. There are two additional steps in this stage.

> a. One thing is to plan, but the second part is to execute. To execute the plan you need to shop for those healthier alternatives and stock up your pantry with those foods.

> b. This might be the sad part; you also need to eliminate the culprits from your pantry. Out of sight, we hope eventually, will be out of mind. To begin with, I found it hard not to have a pack of chips in the pantry. I told myself I would never touch it but I would have it in the pantry just in case I was tempted. This trick never works. Having the culprits and not reaching out to them is harder than you think. It's easier to not have them in the pantry in the first place.

Step 4: Deep examine

This is the stage where you examine the food log and ask yourself a few introspective questions. If you find this step rigorous and overwhelming, go to step 5 and revisit this step.

> ***a. Which foods are partners in crime?*** There are unhealthy foods that get paired with another unhealthy choice. These go hand in hand. For me, it was rice and chips. When I had the urge to eat carbs, I wanted something to go along with it. When I cut out rice, nearly 95% of my chips intake reduced too. Identify the naughty pairs and it's easier than you think, because when you eliminate one, the other one goes too. Sometimes it could be habits. Smoke and coffee or television and ice-cream. Identify these patterns too.

b. What are your moody foods? We all have our comfort foods. Reaching out to them once in a while is fine. Those should not define our lives. Are you eating foods out of boredom, anxiety or mood swings? My go to comfort food during PMS (premenstrual syndrome) was chocolate and desserts.

c. What are your food sources? If you are fuelling your car and your body at the same place, you really need to work on your food sources. Gas stations and convenience stores have the biggest stock of junk foods. Are your sources from fast food places and restaurants? My bag of chips made me crave more of them. The ingredients added to these packaged foods are alarming and the manufacturers aim is for the customers to crave these foods, consume more of them and have a repeat lifelong customer to consume their products.

d. Are your foods well dressed up? Frozen meals, ready to cook items and canned foods, all come well dressed up and neatly packaged and are designed to entice you. Instant meals and microwave culture actually mean inconvenience, in the long term for your health. Identify the method of preparation of your food.

Step 5: Love or fear - what drives you?

> *There are only two driving forces in our life. We choose something or commit to something either out of fear or due to intense love, or sometimes a combination of both.*

I wanted to heal and recover because I wanted to be the best mom, have an abundance of energy and vitality to care for my kids, spend quality time with them and be a great role model. What's your intention? If you are driven by fear, all it takes is to read the first three ingredients that make up the foods you are eating and google them. Are the foods nurturing your body and mind? At the end of the day how do you feel consuming those foods? I felt sluggish, brain fogged, bloated, uneasy, irritable, and constipated when I had unhealthy food choices. I lacked energy and passion throughout the day. Associate these feelings of how you feel or set your intention before reaching out for foods. Revisit step 5 as much as possible throughout the initial stages of your diet elimination and recovery stages.

GUT HEALTH

Understanding about diet, food choices, what to eat, what not to eat, how to eat and when to eat, ultimately has tremendous impact on how the body processes the food inside of it.

The gastrointestinal (GI) track is responsible for the process of digesting the food that comes into our body and ensures that the nutrients from the food are well absorbed and expels the rest. The nutrients absorbed are crucial for the energy production, hormone balance, mental health and skin health. When the body is bombarded with unhealthy food choices or processed foods, the GI track does not recognize the food particles as digestible, and instead it considers them as invaders. This sets off an inflammatory response in our body and it begins to attack these invaders similar to an infection. The gut is also home for trillions of healthy bacteria called the gut microbiome which actually helps to break down the food particles and absorb vital nutrients required for other bodily functions. The bacteria stop growing when they run out of food or are depleted by a heavy ingestion of antibiotics, which is partly the reason for my gut being depleted of the good probiotics.

The other form of depletion to the good bacteria happens through what is called the leaky gut syndrome; inside our gut, we have an extensive intestinal lining covering more than 4,000 square feet of surface area. When working properly, it forms a tight barrier that controls what gets absorbed into the bloodstream. An unhealthy gut lining may have large cracks or holes, allowing partially digested food and toxins to penetrate the tissues beneath it. This may trigger inflammation and changes in the gut flora (normal bacteria) that could lead to problems within the digestive tract and beyond. The good bacteria within the body also keeps the bad bacteria in check, and when there's a good balance of good vs. the bad, the body is said to be in equilibrium. Changes to this equilibrium can cause chronic pains or even autism. An unhealthy balance could cause irritable bowel syndrome (IBS), Crohn's disease or ulcerative colitis. Some kinds of bacteria are considered to be the link between cholesterol and cardio vascular disease or even chronic kidney disease.

With each unhealthy food choice, we tend to confuse the GI track, causing it to attack our own body and not help it to absorb the nutrients, which in turn, causes several physical and mental health issues, and finally, there is too much or too little being expelled at the other end of the spectrum. When digestion is compromised, the body can under produce neurotransmitters like serotonin, which contributes to anxiety, depression and other mental health conditions. It is interesting to note that 95% of serotonin is produced in the small intestine. Scientists call this the gut-brain connection, where the digestive walls have hidden a tiny brain called the enteric nervous system (ENS). The ENS consists of two thin layers of more than a 100 million nerve cells lining your gastrointestinal tract from the esophagus to rectum which is responsible for triggers in emotional shifts, experienced by people coping with irritable bowel syndrome (IBS) and functional bowel problems such as; constipation, diarrhea, bloating, pain and stomach upset. Researchers are finding evidence that irritation in the gastrointestinal system may send signals to the central nervous system (CNS) that trigger mood changes.

> *The first step to improving the gut health is to eliminate the foods that cause an inflammation within our body.*

Avoiding processed foods, alcohol, certain medications and foods that the body is sensitive or allergic to will help improve the gut flora. Also taking probiotics will greatly improve the gut function. The bottom line to having great health lies in the gut. 80-90% of your chronic illness can be alleviated by proper healthy diet.

Step 1: Eliminate foods that cause an inflammation such as processed foods and alcohol completely. Identify the foods that are sensitive or allergic to your body by a food allergy test and eliminate those.

Step 2: Fix nutritional deficiencies with vitamins and supplements.

Step 3: Reintroduce the foods that were eliminated earlier (only the ones that were sensitive or allergic and not the processed foods or alcohol).

ELIMINATION DIET

Eliminating foods can be challenging initially; however, you will begin to notice the benefits quickly which will encourage you to continue along this journey. There are some foods right off the bat that we know are bad, some that may seem healthy might not be the right foods. For example, when I switched from chips to nuts thinking it was healthier, nuts were something I was intolerant to and I continued to have those for a long time without realizing it. Food allergy tests can help reveal which foods are best suited for your body. Every time we consume a food, we are helping our body to heal or to worsen. Each of us have unique needs and the guidelines below are broad based, you might have to choose what is appropriate for you based on discussions with your practitioner. There are so many diet plans that it could be hard to choose one that may suit you. Paleo, Vegan, Gluten-free, Auto Immune Protocol (AIP), Raw foods, Grain-free, Ketogenic Diet, Low Carb Diets, Low Fat diets, Whole 30 and so many more. I did not follow any one particular diet plan; I had to customize it to my needs. 90% of my diet only constitutes of fruits and vegetables now. However, with vegetables, raw salad style did not suit me either - I need to have it cooked, since cold foods don't encourage the digestion process to be efficient. Also being Vegan meant I could not opt for meat sources. When you learn to tune into your body's needs and recognize how the food makes you feel, you can create your own diet that works well for your body. Take baby steps through the process and identify what suits your body. Once your gut and immune system has taken the time to heal by eliminating foods, your body will be able to identify foods that will suit you when you reintroduce them again.

Foods to avoid

- *Gluten:* For anyone with an autoimmune this is the number one thing that needs to be completely eliminated. The proteins found in these foods are inflammatory, can worsen the leaky gut symptoms and even trigger autoimmunity through molecular mimicry. Even with cross contamination, when gluten gets mixed up in foods accidently, I can feel the brain fog symptoms, nausea and diarrhoea right away.

- *Dairy:* butter, buttermilk, cottage cheese, cream, ghee, milk, kefir, sour cream, whey, whipping cream and yogurt

- *Eggs**

- *Beans and Legumes*: black beans, black eyed peas, chickpeas, fava, green, kidney, lentils, lima, mung, navy, peanuts, peas, pinto and soybeans*

- *Refined vegetable oils:* canola, corn, cottonseed oil, palm, peanut, safflower, soybean and sunflower

- *Grains:* amaranth, barley, buckwheat, corn, millet, oats, quinoa, rice, rye, sorghum, spelt and teff*

- *Sweeteners and Sugar:* aspartame, erythritol, mannitol, neotame, saccharin, sorbitol, stevia, sucralose and xylitol

- *Nuts and any butters derived from it:* almonds, brazils, cashews, chestnuts, hazelnuts, macadamia, pecans, pine, pistachios, walnuts*

- *Alcohol*

- *Sodas*

- *Seeds and spices:* anise, caraway, celery seed, chia, cocoa, coffee, coriander, cumin, dill seed, fennel, fenugreek, flax, hemp, mustard, nutmeg, poppy, pumpkin, sesame, sunflower and black pepper*

- *Nightshade family foods:* bell peppers, cayenne, eggplant, goji berries, hot peppers, paprika, potatoes, tomatillos and tomatoes

- *Food Chemicals:* artificial and natural flavors, artificial coloring, carrageenan, guar gum, lecithin, monosodium glutamate (MSG), nitrates and nitrites, phosphoric acid, propylene glycol, trans fats, xantham gum and yeast extract

- *Any names that you don't recognize in the ingredients list*

*some of these can be reintroduced if your gut tolerates it at later stage.

HEALING FOODS TO CONSUME

Choose whole foods with colorful fruits and vegetables, healthy fats, protein and fibrous carbohydrates.

- Green leafy vegetables such as spinach, kale and collard; these are nutrient dense foods that provide antioxidant properties

- Fruits; especially berries, apples and bananas

- A variety of colored vegetables, such as brussel sprouts, broccoli, carrots, beets, and red, yellow, and orange peppers

- Use avocado or olive oils

- Turmeric with curcumin; helps fight inflammation in the body

- Sauerkraut; helps with improving the gut microbiome

- Lean proteins, including tofu, eggs, nuts, beans, and fish

- Fibrous foods, including beans and legumes

- Brain Foods; fatty fish, nuts, dark chocolate, blueberries, beets, avocados, coconut oil, leafy greens and grass fed beef.

NUTRITIONAL DEFICIENCIES

While eliminating foods also make sure you have inadequate nutritionals gaps filled in by vitamins and supplements. Any deficiencies that show up during blood work can be worked out with your practitioner. Below are the medications, vitamins and supplements I take on a daily basis that greatly helped me to recover faster.

Note: Below are to be taken only with advice from medical practitioners as the quality and brand of supplements play a vital role. Some can be harmful if proper precautions and adequate dosage levels are not followed.

4:00 a.m. – Thyroid medication T4 and T3 Levothyroxine and Liothyronine on an empty stomach. *Note after taking the medica-*

tion its best to wait for an hour before eating any food.

For 8 weeks during the elimination diet my ND had recommended L-glutathione forte that needs to be mixed with one glass of water and taken on an empty stomach. I used to keep a cup with one spoon of this powder by my bedside and mix with a glass of water, stir it and use it to take my thyroid medications in the morning.

8:30 a.m. – after breakfast I take my Probiotics, vitamin c, zinc 30 picolinate and methylcobalamin B12 - a chewable form that needs to be placed under the tongue and it gets dissolved by itself. *Note the first dose of vitamins needs to be taken at least 4 hours after the thyroid medication so there is no interference with the supplements.*

12:30 p.m. – before lunch I take digestive enzyme and after lunch I take multivitamin, omega 3 (vegetarian options are available too), vitamin d 4000 IU and selenium 200mg.

2:30 p.m. – another dose of T3 Liothyronine medicine. My ND had split the dose between morning and evening so I had sustained energy levels throughout the day. *Note this needs to be taken two hours after lunch with nothing being consumed during that 2-hour period.*

3:30 p.m. – after 30 minutes of taking T3 you may have your evening snacks. I had celery juice for a few months. I was recommended to have that every day if possible.

6:00 p.m. – after dinner I take vitamin c, probiotics, magnesium citrate (helps with constipation or use Magnesium Glycinate), biotin and vitamin A. Having an early dinner also helps to follow an intermittent fasting.

> **Intermittent fasting is where you give your body a fasting period so you can better utilize the energy levels.**

When your body is constantly working on digesting food, the body's energy reserves are directed towards that function. Intermittent fasting helps stabilize the blood sugar levels, reduces inflammation and stress, decreases blood pressure and cholesterol levels and improves resting heart rate and brain health.

REINTRODUCING FOODS

The good news is that the elimination diet is not forever. I followed an eight-week plan. Some plans could be for 90 days as well. Go slowly with reintroducing foods - my ND had suggested that I begin with foods that have a low ranking next to it—begin with 1, then move to 2 and then finally introduce 3. The levels 1-3 denote the intensity of allergy or sensitivities. Begin with one and consume that food for 3 days. Make note of any changes or symptoms you may see. Then move onto the next food item and try it for a few days and make a note of it. Although this process seems long drawn, it eventually benefits your body and provides you great peace of mind that you are consuming only the foods that suit your body. As soon as you eliminate the foods that don't suit you, you will notice your energy levels will peak, you will feel lighter and have greater mental clarity. Your body will seem more flexible and your mood will be much happier. While reintroducing foods, if you experience headaches, bloating, uneasiness, constipation, hives or nausea, these are symptoms that your body is not yet ready to accept the reintroduction. You may wait for a few more days and try again.

MOTTOS ON MY PLATE

- I use Himalayan Pink Salt instead of regular salt since it contains more trace minerals.

- Avoid Teflon's and non-stick cookware, instead opt for cast iron cookware or stainless steel. When the non-stick cookware or Teflon's are overheated while cooking, they produce fumes which cause people to experience flu like symptoms. With repeated heating and cooling, the Teflon's can also produce harmful PFOA (perfluorooctanoic acid) that can even leach into food.

- Avoid plastic spatulas, similarly, they can cause a release of harmful chemicals during high heat. Avoid plastic storage containers to store foods as these plastics contain Bisphenol A (BPA), a chemical that, once ingested, mimics estrogen in our bodies.

- I plan the cooking menu for the entire week and make a list of the items to buy and shop once a week. It saves money, time and energy.

- I take a few hours during the weekend to cut the vegetables to cook for the week ahead which saves a lot of time during weekdays.

- I use Olive and Avocado oils to cook for myself and Coconut oil for my family at times.

- I have an early dinner before 6pm and have my next meal the following day at 8am. I have 14 hours of intermittent fasting for my body to benefit from.

- I use turmeric with curcumin as well as ginger in my everyday cooking, which helps fight inflammation in the body and boosts my immunity as well.

- I use different herbs like mint which helps with digestions and cilantro helps with detox to garnish my meals.

- As soon as I wake up I drink a glass of warm water on an empty stomach. I have warm water right after lunch and dinner too. It helps with digestion and avoids bloating and uneasiness after meals. Also a brisk walk for a few minutes after meals will help with digestion.

- I drink good filtered water throughout the day to keep myself well hydrated.

- I always carry snacks in my bag so I don't end up buying something outside out of desperation that I would regret later. Also keep your medications handy in the bag so you don't end up skipping or taking it on time.
- Never count your calorie or your salary, both lead to agony!

What's your MOTTO?

CHECK-IN

1. What does your daily diet look like?
_____
_____

2. How do you feel after consuming foods? Note down how your body feels after breakfast, lunch, dinner or snacks.
_____
_____

3. Maintain a food log to determine what foods you need to eliminate from your diet. Refer to the Diet Roadmap to help you in your journey.
_____
_____

4. What is your number one concern when it comes to having a healthy diet?
_____
_____

5. How would you like to feel at the end of the day? After a few weeks? After a few months?
_____
_____

6. Consult with your physician or nutritionist to identify nutritional deficiencies. If required, go in for a food allergy/intolerance test.
_____
_____

SUMMARY

• One of the most important things we can do for our health is to eat wisely every day. 'Food is medicine' when consumed properly.

• Begin with making note of what you consume, identify foods that are unhealthy, plan your replacement options, examine the sources of food and get clear on your intention to heal.

• Understanding about diet, food choices, what to eat, what not to eat and how to eat, ultimately has tremendous impact on how the body processes the food inside.

• The gut is home for trillions of healthy bacteria called the gut microbiome which actually helps to break down the food particles and absorb vital nutrients required for other bodily functions.

• The bottom line to having great health lies in the gut. 80-90% of your chronic illness can be alleviated by proper healthy diet.

• The first step to improving the gut health is to eliminate the foods that cause an inflammation within our body.

• Fix nutritional deficiencies by taking in additional supplements that your body might be lacking.

• Each of us have unique needs and dietary patterns, take baby steps through the process of identifying and consuming delicious healthy foods that nurture your body.

CHAPTER ELEVEN

THE MARMA MOTTO

Over 3000 years ago, the Ayurvedic practitioners knew the secret to detoxify, strengthen and revitalize the body. Ayurveda is an ancient holistic system developed in India. The Ayurvedic practitioners knew that when certain points of our body are inflicted, they could cause serious damage to our health, or even death, but when taken care of, they could provide deep, enriching physical, mental and emotional benefits. These secret points were called the Marma, which are vital points of the body that contain prana or energy. The word Marma, is of Sanskrit origin, which means secret or hidden. A marma is the junction point of physiology and consciousness, where two or more types of tissues meet; it could be tissues, veins, ligaments, bones or joints.

> *The Ayurvedic practitioners developed Marma Therapy as one of the most powerful healing modalities for stress and pain management.*

The therapy is a specialized massage technique that is useful to heal the damaged tissue, to detoxify by activating the lymphatic system, stimulates the function of internal organs and unblocks the tension from the nerves, muscles and joints, thereby unblocking the energy flow or the prana within the body.

The secret power of these energy centers is that when stimulated, they release a steady stream of prana to restore balance in the body. Ayurveda says that in order to be healthy, we must allow vital energy or prana to flow smoothly. If we are in imbalance and get carried away by lifestyle or thoughts that are detrimental to our lives, this energy is blocked and the prana cannot flow properly, therefore the body does not function harmoniously.

BENEFITS OF MARMA THERAPY

- Provides detoxification of mind, body and spirit

- Prevents aging

- Releases deep tension in muscles

- Enhances sleep quality

- Provides tissue regeneration

- Helps minimize asthma and anxiety

- Clears troubled emotions and psychological blockages

- Improves circulation and energy flow

- Helps with migraine headaches and chronic pains

- Minimizes hyper tension

- Relieves muscle pain, stiffness in the joints, and any restriction on body movement that may result from too much or too little exercise

MARMA ABHYANGA

Abhyanga is an Ayurveda method of oil massage with marma therapy. Gentle pressure on the marma points while performing massage gives prana energy to the body and mind which provides the ultimate healing. Special herb infused ayurvedic oil is slowly warmed up and massaged into the skin. The massage is deeply relaxing, detoxifies, strengthens and rejuvenates the entire body. It calms and strengthens the central nervous system, improves the lymph flow and stimulates the nervous system. For Hashimoto's, the Abhyanga is extremely beneficial and helps with fatigue, dry skin, balances the hormones and minimizes painful menstruation, improves digestive disorders, insomnia, irritable bowel syndrome (IBS), joint pains and minimizes visible signs of aging. Although a visit to an Ayurvedic practitioner or massage therapist would be beneficial, you can also do it at home on a weekly basis. My mom used to give me oil massages every week when I was a baby. Baby oil massage is an ancient custom practiced in India even to this day. These rituals have been practiced and passed down for hundreds of generations. I continue this ritual until this day and also do the massages for my kids. When I skip a week with my personal massage or for my kids, I find that something major is missing in my life! I feel rejuvenated, uplifted and energized with these weekly rituals.

TIPS ON HOW TO DO ABYANGA AT HOME

• Choose a day where you can dedicate some time for the massage once a week. I choose Fridays. It takes 60-90 minutes depending on how long you prefer it to be. You need to ensure you have the time and don't feel rushed through the process.

• You can choose any oil like almond, olive, sesame or coconut. Almond oil soaks into the skin quickly and is an excellent moisturizer with antifungal properties. Olive oil helps provide relief from inflammation, aches and muscle spasms. Sesame oil is thick and may leave the skin oily, it can be blended with other lighter oils and has a distinct aroma. I use coconut oil since it provides deep hydration and has anti-bacterial and anti-fungal properties. The fatty acids in the oil help to kill the harmful pathogens including viruses and fungi and helps prevent infections. It also acts as a good hair conditioner and helps reduce frizz.

- You may also add some essential oils to the diffuser or blend them with any of the oils mentioned above. Make sure the oils are pure and of a high grade quality so you get the maximum benefits while using it.

1. Lemongrass: helps detox the thyroid while maintaining its natural lymphatic function. It has powerful anti-fungal and anti-inflammatory properties and can assist the cells that are associated with rebuilding damaged tissues. It can also be applied to swollen or inflamed thyroid area because this area is in need of repair. Lemongrass oil can promote healthy circulation and nervous system responses.

2. Frankincense: has immune boosting, anti-inflammatory and pain relieving properties. It protects the thyroid by destroying the free radicals in the body. This needs to be mixed with base oil and applied to the thyroid area. Supporting your health at a cellular level, Frankincense boosts immune function to help bridge the gap from hormones to the thyroid and normalizes your body functions. It can also help with dull and dry skin that are common with thyroid issues.

3. Clove: clove essential oil helps regulate your body's stress response. This oil has a warm scent and brings a calming effect immediately. The main constituent of clove oil, eugenol, can really help your body fend off environmental toxins and detox through free radicals, as well as giving that immune system a healthy boost.

4. Myrrh: has great anti-inflammatory properties and is an anti-oxidant helping your body to filter out the toxins. Myrrh essential oil, not only benefits your skin but also supports healthy emotions and boosts the immune system. Your body synthesizes chemicals called cytokines, which play a major role in the progression of autoimmune thyroid diseases. A great benefit of myrrh is that it can keep your cells from producing this chemical, potentially thwarting your body's attack on your thyroid gland.

5. *Peppermint*: helps with digestion, reduces nausea, boosts sluggish metabolism. Energizing and refreshing to your mood and mental state, peppermint not only fights that overwhelming fatigue but also supports healthy digestion. Peppermint is a powerful oil that affects your central nervous system and your cells' abilities to be stimulated, which could help rev up your underactive thyroid if you are dealing with hypothyroidism. It brings immediate cooling effects and can be helpful to use during hot flushes.

6. *Rose geranium*: has anti-inflammatory properties and helps with an underactive thyroid. This may be applied topically on the neck area near the thyroid. It also helps with anxiety.

- Warm the oil gently by placing the bottle of oil in warm water; using cotton balls, begin to apply the oil to the scalp. Partition the hair in small segments to make sure the oil reaches the scalp.

- Begin by gently massaging the scalp in circular motions, especially above and around the ear lobes, back of the head at the base of your skull and proceed to massage all over the face, neck and body.

- Make sure the oil is warm throughout while massaging all over the body. Massage clockwise near the belly area which helps improve digestion.

- Start from the top of your head and move to the legs. Massaging the ear lobes, palms and bottom of the feet helps to deeply relax your mind and body.

• You may adopt long strokes, kneading, tapping or applying pressure with your fingertips along the skin; choose whichever comes easy for you.

• Once done you will notice most of the oil has been absorbed into your skin, later wash your hair and body using mild soap to make sure you don't remove all of the oil from your hair and skin. Throughout the day, by retaining the oil on your body it helps to provide deep moisturizing benefits.

After the Abhyanga session you will experience excessive hunger and a restorative, relaxing night's sleep. During massage there is release of serotonin which is helpful in the production of melatonin, which helps regulate the circadian rhythm. Also it helps to reduce the cortisol levels and increases the oxytocin and even dopamine levels. Cortisol is a stress hormone that supports your "fight-or-flight" response. When your body is exposed to it long-term, you may experience anxiety, depression, sleep problems, weight gain, and even heart disease. Oxytocin, on the other hand, is known as the "love" hormone. I usually go to bed early that night and wake up rejuvenated and energized the next day. You might tend to not feel sleepy right away or not feel rejuvenated the following day, which is totally normal too, but you will feel hungry for sure.

> *Once you begin to have these regular mini spas at home, you will have a noticeably higher quality of sleep and experience the amazing power of restorative night rest.*

SLEEP

Sleep is one of the most delicious five letter words and one of my love languages. I've had a long history with lots of sleep and a lack of sleep. As a child I used to nap for 3-4 hours in the afternoon and also manage to sleep for 10-11 hours at night. Summer holidays were easy on my parents since I used to take my naps or sleep a lot and they did not have to take care of me much, except for providing me with lunch and dinner (I used to skip my breakfast time sleeping too). During my early 20s when I began my career in marketing, the advertisements had to be released to the newspapers by 12 noon and I felt it was too early a deadline! When I was pregnant with my first child, the tables turned and I was experiencing interruptions in my sleep for the first time in my life. Tossing and turning on the bed with big belly or waking up for restroom breaks were new to me. Then when my son was born, he was colicky and night time feedings kept me awake for most part. By the time things settled with the first, I was pregnant again and the whole story repeated itself. So the first taste of interrupted sleep began with pregnancy and continued for several years.

> **Later being diagnosed with Hashimoto's, sleep became the most looked forward to and the most difficult activity to accomplish.**

When you are hypothyroid you long to sleep and no amount of sleep will rejuvenate you, when you are hyperthyroid, anxiety, heart palpitations, night sweats and racing thoughts are sure to keep one awake the whole night. During one of my doctor's visits I even mentioned that I wished I could go on a vacation all by myself and just sleep. I would imagine of days of having to do nothing. I had been on both ends of the spectrum with too much sleep during my early years of my life, to too little sleep during the motherhood days. Both are equally bad, a balance is crucial for optimal health. Too much sleep would make you lethargic and unproductive since you have little time to accomplish the things you want to in a day. Too little sleep would create the undesired version of yourself by making you angry, irritated and short tempered, long term it could cause weight gain, increased risk of heart disease, high blood pressure, diabetes, kidney problems, a decrease in immunity and even a stroke.

I learnt to get into deep sleep and feel rejuvenated with 8 hours of sleep. The period in my life where I missed restful nights, I learnt never to take sleep for granted and I'm in awe of the fine balance with sleep and wakefulness. When you don't snooze you lose - sleep deficit impairs your learning and information retaining ability leading to memory loss. Matthew Walker is a British Researcher and in his TEDx Talks mentions about how researchers have found that there are big and powerful brainwaves that happen during one's deepest sleep stages, and there are bursts of electrical activity which are produced called sleep spindles. The combination of deep sleep brain waves with the sleep spindles, act as a file transfer mechanism at night. Similar to a computer moving its files to storage, the brain makes sure the memory is transferred from the short-term retention to long term retention zone, and protecting them. Learning faculties and memory retention are crucial aspects that are determined by sleep.

Walker also points out another most interesting study which brings out the correlation between sleep loss and immune system.

The immune cell activity reduces by 70% when sleep is reduced to 4 hours in one single night.

The drastic immune deficiency is caused not by loss of sleep over several nights, it's one single night! Which means your body is more susceptible to numerous forms of cancer (bowel, prostrate and breast) with loss of sleep. The World Health Organization has even categorized any form of night-shift work as a form of carcinogen due to the disruption with your circadian rhythm cycle. Lack of sleep even impacts your DNA genetic code; researchers found that 711 genes were impacted by reducing the sleep to 6 hours a night instead of 8 hours. The genes that were impacted were associated with immune deficiency, promotion of tumors, long-term chronic inflammation within the body, stress and as a result, cardio vascular disease. Sleep is of paramount importance to your overall wellbeing.

TIPS FOR BETTER SLEEP

• During the day, spend time outside in the sunlight for a few hours so your body automatically regulates the circadian rhythm.

• Avoid heavy meals, sugary foods, caffeine and alcohol before bedtime. I take my magnesium supplements after dinner which helps me fall asleep faster. Avoid relying on sleep supplements on a long-term basis.

• Adequate exercise during the day or walking during the evenings will help you sleep as soon as you hit your bed.

• Meditations right before bedtime will help with the quality of your sleep, with deep inhale and exhale actions, it allows the body to sink deeper into sleep (see more on meditations in the Zen MOTTO section).

• Maintain a regular sleep and wake up time. Going to bed before 10pm helps your body not to experience the second burst of energy which will keep you awake much longer. Wake up before sunrise so your body is in tune with the nature's wake up and sleep cycles.

• A warm shower, reading a book, listening to relaxing music, calming teas and lotions or essential oils will help your body ease into sleep. I apply lotion and massage my palms and feet at night to reduce stress and anxiety before I sleep.

• I watch short funny videos every evening and turn my phone on 'dark until sunlight' mode (night time mode) which reduces the bright light from the phone, I dim the lights at least an hour before bedtime and avoid digital devices before bedtime (see more on the Digital Sunset MOTTO).

The Body MOTTO has 4 key components – good exercise, healthy diet, yoga - the link between your mind and body, and the last one is rest. The circle is not complete without rest and relaxation. Our body goes through different sleep cycles at night and produces different brain wave patterns. The Alpha brain waves happens right before and during sleep and deep calm. The Beta brain waves are associated with memory, cognitive abilities and alertness. These are produced all day while at work or any activity. The Delta brain waves occur during deep sleep while the Theta brain waves which are higher up in the frequency scale, are associated with deep emotion and creative ideas. The Gamma brain waves have the highest frequency and occur during stages of extreme happiness and they help with absorbing new information. The Alpha and Gamma waves are produced during meditation. Buddhist monks and experienced meditators can get into the super special frequency of gamma waves which are associated with robust brain function.

Good rest leads to a wakeful and productive mind. The next section we delve into the power of mindfulness.

What's your MOTTO?

CHECK-IN

1. Do you feel well rested and rejuvenated every day?
_____
_____

2. How many hours of sleep do you get every day?
_____
_____

3. Is your mind able to mentally switch off and do you get to sleep as soon as you hit the bed?
_____
_____

4. If you feel your sleep is disrupted at nights - how often and why?
_____
_____

5. What is your number one concern when it comes to rest/sleep? (work hours, disruptions, other unhealthy life style habits?)
_____
_____

6. What is one thing you would like to change about the way you rest? (increase or decrease sleep hours, go to bed on time, wake up early, etc.)
_____
_____

SUMMARY

- The secret points in the body are called the Marma, which are vital points that contain prana or energy.

- Abhyanga is an Ayurveda way of oil massage with marma therapy. Gentle pressure on the marma points while doing massage gives prana energy to the body and mind which gives ultimate healing.

- For Hashimoto's, the Abhyanga is extremely beneficial and helps with fatigue, dry skin, balances the hormones and minimizes painful menstruation, improves digestive disorders, insomnia, irritable bowel syndrome (IBS), joint pains and minimizes visible signs of aging.

- Researchers found correlation between sleep loss and the immune system. The immune cell activity reduces by 70% when sleep is reduced to 4 hours in one single night. The drastic immune deficiency is caused not by loss of sleep over several nights, it's one single night!

- Good rest leads to a wakeful and productive mind.

THE MIND MOTTO

Nature and all beings are governed by a universal law of causation, which means that every action has a root cause that defines it and initiates it. As humans we make decisions every single day, each has its own cause and the effects that go with it. We are all made up of matter which comprises of the body, the mind and the intellect. The body is the physical manifestation of our organs; the mind is where the preferences - likes, dislikes and emotions are stored. The intellect is where the reasoning capabilities rest, it's the mature part of the brain that can help make decisions based on the knowledge and wisdom it has garnered over the years.

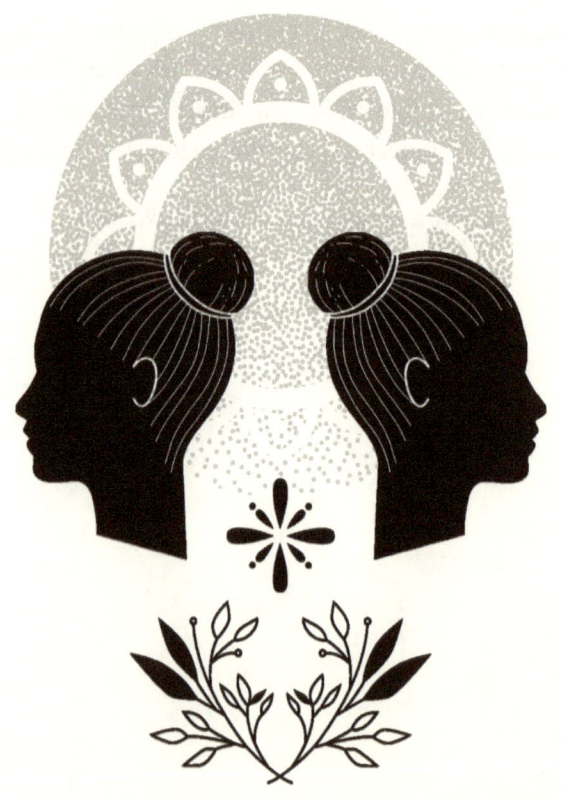

When impulsive decisions are made by the mind, the intellect is what makes you stop in your tracks and question the motive to make that decision. When the mind takes over, the rationale and objective is being clouded by emotions and desires. To know if you are ruled by your mind or your intellect, simply look into your feelings and observe how you feel. When decisions are made using the mind, you involve your senses and give in to your emotions which might lead to regrets later, when decisions are made by the intellect, there is peace, steadiness and calmness and less regret later. Strengthening the intellect and protecting it from negativity becomes crucial to lead an intentional life. The Mind MOTTO will lead you through the process of gaining control over the intellect through –The Zen MOTTO, The Hola MOTTO, The Digital Sunset MOTTO and The Reasoning MOTTO.

CHAPTER TWELVE

THE ZEN MOTTO

Meditation is training your mind to focus and bringing the awareness to your breath. Although it sounds simple to sit and focus on your breath, it can be a challenge to see how the mind gets caught up with several thoughts. A thoughtless mind seems to be daunting and the more you focus on not thinking, the more you end up thinking. A thoughtless state cannot be achieved however with practice, instead we learn not to react to our thoughts. The first good sign is when you notice your thoughts, which mean the awareness of the thought has come up. We simply observe our thoughts and let it pass by our mind like clouds floating away in the sky without getting attached to those thoughts and bring the awareness back to our breath. Sometimes there could be moments where there are simply no thoughts, where your mind slips into total tranquility for a few seconds, as soon as we realize that, we tend to have the thoughts back. With practice and dedication, we learn to exercise the elasticity of the mind by stretching the space or the time gap between our thoughts so we can get to experience the tranquility longer.

I had never attended any meditation classes nor did I even know what exactly meditation was when I got started. After I had quit my job, I used to begin my day listening to some relaxing music, did some yoga and towards the end, I sat down quietly for 5 minutes. What started as a simple practice grew stronger and I continued to practice it regularly every single day. I had learnt some pranayama's which is synchronizing the breath and having control over it when I was in my early 20s. As explained in the Yogic MOTTO, prana is the life force and ayama means control. With practicing the only two pranayama's that I had learnt, and sitting quietly for 5 minutes, I began to observe how slow my breathing was and the calming effect it had on me. Over time I could sit down to meditate for at least 20 minutes. When the time span gradually increased, my kids would wake up and come over to my room where I meditated and jump onto my lap with a thud, and my meditation would abruptly come to an end. This happened for a few days and I disliked the fact that I could not ease out of meditation and have a smooth finish to my practice. The only solution I realized was to wake up much earlier than what I was used to. One good habit initiated another great habit in my life. I began to wake up at 5am, which would have been an ungodly hour to wake up 15 years ago for me. I enjoyed the feeling of staying in meditation for longer and it drove me to even wake up early, getting to know more about myself was a priority and I made the time for it. This was the biggest turning point in my life, the early mornings gave the extra oomph to the meditations and my practice was much longer for more than 30 minutes every single day. I began to see meditation as a way to recharge my battery every day. During the beginning stages, there were some days I might have more activities that would drain my charged energy quicker, but

> *I noticed I was not totally falling apart or reacting to events, I was able to combat the stress and knew I was building a foundation for personal wellness.*

Meditation takes patience and time. It's called practicing meditation for a reason since we can never claim to have an accomplished status, there's always more to learn and know more about. Some people tend to get frustrated and sometimes even angry or bored with their first attempt. It could be challenging if we are trying to monitor and remove every single thought. Also not getting too attached to the results will make meditations more experiential. Most research shows that meditations can work quickly in a short period of time. It's best not to use analytics or ask what's the goal? Am I progressing? Or am I doing it the right way? You may observe how you feel at the end of a session to know the impact of meditation and how you are progressing. If you feel calmer, relaxed, happy, blissful, energized, rejuvenated or at times, even sleepy, since that is your body's way of asking you to take the needed rest, then you are progressing. You will feel less stressed (when stressed your breath is shallow, when relaxed you tend to take slow long breaths), more accepting and at greater peace during the initial stages. If you continue to return to your mat for meditation everyday then that's a great sign. Over time the effects may continue in all other areas of your life too, you may become less judgmental on other's behaviors and actions, more compassionate, have greater mental clarity and decision making abilities, develop a sense of urgency as well as the courage to work on your purpose, gain a sense of responsibility towards your health and wellbeing, begin to eat healthy, become more intuitive and feel a strong sense of inner guidance and be more aware of your actions, thoughts and words.

Think of meditation as peeling an onion. We have to peel away the layers of distractions and what we are made of to get to the core, sometimes even causing tears.

> ***Meditation is simply removing the distractions and the exterior made up identities to get to our true inner core.***

Once we reach that place, going through the process of peeling, the core onion can help make our lives more flavorful. True healing comes from peeling and going through the process. Enrolling in a class and having a teacher to guide you through the process could be beneficial if you find it overwhelming to do it on your own.

BEGINNER TIPS FOR MEDITATION

• *Zen Spot:* Find a quiet place in your home where you can meditate. You may choose a specific corner in your home intended only for meditation.

• *Zen Time:* Choose a convenient time you can meditate where your distractions might be less and make sure you get to do it the same time every day. The ideal times are early mornings (start during sunrise or right before sunrise) and evenings (during sunset) or before bedtime (read more in the Golden Hour MOTTO section.) I meditate early mornings and right before bedtime which greatly improved my sleep. During the day I take a few deep breaths to calm the mind and body. Increasing the frequency of meditation sessions helps to calm down your body and recharge your energies throughout the day.

• *Zen Props:* A cushion or a blanket to make you more comfortable. I also use a scarf to cover up my eyes. When you close your eyes, you turn off the visual distractions and you get enhanced abilities on other senses and sensations, you take your experience to a whole new dimension. I sometimes place a cool towel on the inside of the scarf which makes me feel refreshed and rejuvenated after the meditation. Some meditators also adopt an open eye meditation focusing on a candle light or an object however personally I have not tried this.

• *Zen Pose:* There are a few poses to adopt when seated on the floor, you may also sit on a chair if you have any trouble sitting down. Some of the poses are; **Lotus pose** with legs overlapped over the other and palms facing upward, **Japanese posture** if your legs and hips allow and if it's comfortable and **Padmasana or Sukhasana** where the legs are not overlapped but more at ease like the criss cross applesauce pose, and this is the way Indians sit on the floor to eat. I personally do the lotus pose or sometimes the Japanese pose or both. I feel more grounded with the lotus posture, however for a very long duration my legs go numb in this posture. If sitting poses don't suit you well, you can choose the corpse pose which is **Savasana**. I personally do not try to meditate in this pose as I tend to sleep right away. However, I do this for few minutes after my yoga practice to settle down and calm my body.

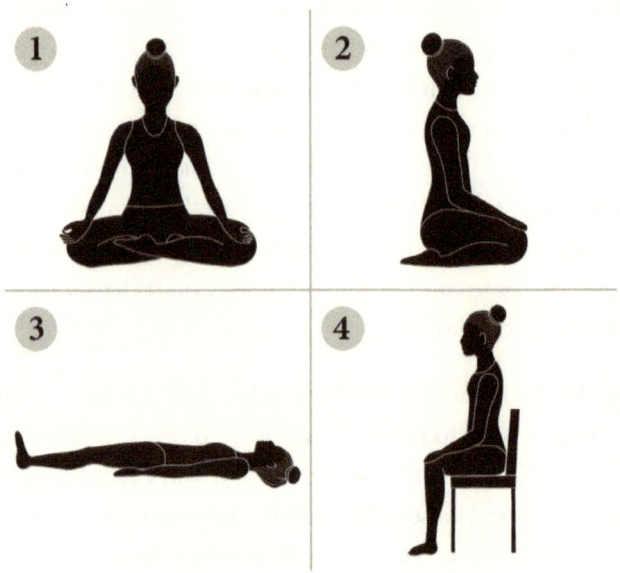

1- Lotus 2- Japanese 3- Corpse 4- Chair

• *Zen Posture:* When seated make sure your spine is erect, you are able to sit upright and not hunched over. Maintain good posture, one which is comfortable and can be maintained for a long time. The spine is the conductor of energies and how we conduct the energy depends on the erectness of our spine. One Yogic guru says the spine is the axis of the universe. Meaning we can channelize our energies from our spine and through to all other parts of the body.

• *Zen Gesture or Mudra:* You may use a hand gesture or mudras to channel your body's energy flow. Chakras are the circular vortexes of energy that are placed in seven different points on the spinal column, and all the seven chakras are connected to the various organs and glands within the body. These chakras are responsible for distributing the life energy, which is also known as Qi or Prana. The throat chakra governs the thyroid, parathyroid and respiratory system. The **Akash Mudra** helps to activate the throat chakra. To form this mudra, bring your thumb and middle finger to touch each other gently, do not use force or pressure to press down the finger. This is a popular mudra and helps with concentration, eliminating negative thoughts and congestion, regularizes the heart beat and helps with blood pressure. Through use of breath, focus and mudra, we are working on channelizing the energy within our body. There are several mudras, however as a beginner, open palms rested on the lap can also be used in place of a mudra.

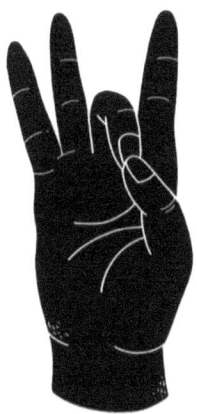

Akash Mudra

- ***Zen Mantra:*** The mantra associated with the Throat Chakra is HAM (pronounced HUM). Chanting this mantra will work to remove the blockages in the throat chakra that prevent it from moving through to the other main chakras. I chant OM before, during and after my meditation. One way to feel the vibration more within your body is to close your ears with your thumb and place the other fingers on the center of the forehead and closed eyes and chant OM extending the M sound to reverberate more. With practice you will begin to notice the vibrations near the heart and also get to feel it within your head and throat. The mantras can be used during grounding poses in yoga such as the garland pose or mountain poses to enhance the experience (refer to The Yogic MOTTO for these poses).

BEFORE MEDITATION

Yogic gurus and ancient teachings say that taking a cold shower before yoga or meditation is really beneficial. A cold shower increases your mental alertness, stimulates the anti-depression hormones and accelerates your metabolism. I begin with a few stretches, listening to calming music and do a **Super Brain Yoga** to increase the brain capacity.

- *Super Brain Yoga:* Place the arms crisscrossed in front of your chest and hold onto the opposite ear lobes while doing squats, this is believed to make you smarter. Research has showed that this helps with autism, attention deficit and behavioural issues too. Chinese acupuncturists and Indian yogis believe the ear lobes contain energy meridians to points in the brain and pineal gland. The super brain activates the brain's energy connections. The right lobe activates the left brain and vice versa. Gently massaging the ear lobe activates the pineal gland which regulates the circadian rhythm, reduces mental stress, and improves overall mood and well-being.

- *Pranayamas:* I practice the **Sitali pranayama**, open your mouth and roll your tongue. Begin to take in deep breaths through your tongue and exhale through the nose. This helps to cool down your body, expels toxins and has an immediate calming effect to your mind. Another excellent preparation for meditation is the **Alternate Nostril Breathing** or the Nadi Shodhana. It involves inhaling through one nostril and exhaling through the other. Bring the right hand up to the nose and fold the index and middle fingers to the palm, so that you can use the thumb to close the right nostril, and the ring finger to close the left nostril. Be sure that you are not bending over to bring the head down to your hand. Continue to alternate with inhaling through the right nostril for 3 counts and exhaling to the left for 6 counts. Gradually increase to 4 and 8 counts; 5 and 10 counts. Now begin to inhale 3 counts on the left nostril and exhale to 6 counts. When inhaling or exhaling, only one nostril is open and the other one remains closed. Through this practice we are circulating the energy within the body and this has tremendous benefits when done correctly and regularly.

DURING MEDITATION

You begin to calm down and focus on your breath or candle light (if your eyes are open). I personally close my eyes with a scarf and focus or point my eyes in between my brows or the third eye. This might be uncomfortable initially, however you may get used to it with practice. You may continue to focus on breathing and not focus on the third eye too. These are variations to the focus point, take it slowly and see which method is comfortable for you or comes more intuitively for you. You may also focus on a mantra or music if breath or eye does not work for you. There are also guided meditations available where the process is to do a mental body scan of the different parts of your body. The whole idea is to exercise the brain muscles for increasing the attention span and focus.

By focusing on the moment we can get to the true essence of meditation. There is no good or bad meditation, even a few minutes of the worst meditation (as per your version) is much better than no meditation. There is a Zen proverb that 'you should sit in meditation for twenty minutes every day - unless you are too busy; then you should sit for an hour.' **I feel meditation is something that even if you feel you are failing, you are still winning with your personal wellbeing.**

What's your MOTTO?

CHECK-IN

1. Have you tried to meditate before? If yes, how was your experience?

_____
_____
_____
_____

2. What is one thing that is stopping you from getting started on meditation? (lack of interest, lack of time, seems too complex, not sure how to do, etc?)

_____
_____
_____
_____

3. How can you overcome your concern of not getting started? (by joining a class, self-learning from videos, ask a friend or family member to help you)

_____
_____
_____
_____

SUMMARY

- Meditation is training your mind to focus and bringing the awareness to your breath.

- The first good sign is when you notice your thoughts, which mean the awareness of the thought has come up.

- Not getting too attached to the results will make meditations more experiential.

- Think of meditation as peeling an onion. We have to peel the layers of distractions and what we are made of to get to the core, sometimes even causing tears. Meditation is simply removing the distractions and the exterior made up identities to reach our true inner core. Once we get there, going through the process of peeling, the core onion can help make our lives more flavorful.

- There is no good or bad meditation, even a few minutes of your worst meditation (as per your version) is much better than no meditation.

- Meditation is something that even if you feel you are failing, you are still winning with your personal wellbeing.

CHAPTER THIRTEEN

THE HOLA MOTTO

During the initial stages of my illness, a general physician once mentioned that it was all in my head. It's ironic because not only were the symptoms that I experienced for real, and not imaginary ones, the truth that gradually revealed itself was that I had nothing left in my head. My mental faculties were dimmed—I lacked clarity and reasoning which was due to brain fog, a symptom of Hashimoto's. I felt like a zombie for the most part, the constant fatigue and longing to sleep made it worse. My attention span decreased, I would read and reread pages in a book and still be unable to comprehend it. Reading for a while or working where it involved some attention, left me drained, wiped out and I would sleep for hours to recover from it. My thoughts were clouded and no amount of sleep would make me feel rejuvenated. I could sense that simple tasks were becoming more of a challenge. When I could not remember my daughter's year of birth one day, it hit me like ton of bricks. I knew I was experiencing some serious forgetfulness. When driving, even with the GPS, I would get lost. I was once so lost I called my husband to ask how I could get back home. He asked me where exactly I was and I screamed back on the phone saying "I'm lost and I don't know where I am."

Although to this day we laugh over that incident, the truth of the matter is Hashimoto's can really result in your mind getting lost and not knowing where to look for it. I used to use the compass on my phone while at home to see which way was north, south, east and west. I would then turn around a few times and ask myself which direction I faced now, I wouldn't be able to tell.

> *Mental health is one of the most ignored aspects in Hashimoto's. Learn to identify the symptoms early on so you can take action right away.*

Symptoms of brain fog

- Forgetfulness
- Shorter attention span
- Brain fatigue – even simple brain tasks would cause extreme fatigue and sleepiness
- Difficulty making decisions
- Poor concentration
- Difficulty learning new information
- Lack of attention and interest

You might look and act normal to others; however, you might constantly be in a state of fuzziness. You might have trouble expressing your thoughts through words and making meaningful sentences, since you have to think through every word from your memory to your mouth without the disruption. Sometimes you might look lost or spaced out but your processor is actually working on slower mode and others might mistakenly think you are disinterested in them or the conversation. You might forget what you wanted to say mid-sentence or not know why you entered a room or what you were about to do. Expressing yourself might be the hardest thing to do. If any of these sound familiar, then you're not alone. Behind the scenes however this is what is happening to your thyroid, brain and body.

The thyroid is a powerhouse that controls every single action in your body. The thyroid gland is responsible for the hormones that have tremendous influence on your body. With Hashimoto's the thyroid is unable to produce the adequate levels of different hormones which causes multiple disruptions to the working of the body. The estrogen which is a powerful sex hormone is affected causing a drop in the levels. When the levels drop it could mean fluctuations in the menstrual cycle, or menopause. However, another crucial role that estrogen plays is in the optimal brain functioning, regulating the cognition and body temperature. The hormones act as anti-inflammatory agents in the brain reducing the number of brain immune cells. When the estrogen levels drop, the immune cells are not under check thereby causing an increase in the inflammation. **Estrogens influence the immune and inflammatory processes and also reveal a higher rate of autoimmune diseases in women.** When estrogen levels are in excess, it could cause problems in blood sugar levels (insulin resistance) and can disrupt the hormone leptin, which provides a feeling of fullness therefore which leads to obesity. With thyroid condition, the neurotransmitters in the brain are also affected. Neurotransmitters are a type of chemical messenger the nervous system uses as a way to communicate and provide directions and control to the rest of the body. Acetylcholine - a crucial neurotransmitter for learning, memory, and menopause - is affected due to the thyroid causing low acetylcholine levels which causes brain fog. With a healthy diet (refer to The Plateful MOTTO on healthy brain foods), exercise (refer to The Moto MOTTO and The Zen MOTTO on Super Brain Yoga) and proper sleep, these can however be regularized. Some of the other brain exercises that can help reverse or minimize the brain fog levels are listed below.

SUPER BRAIN EXERCISES

> *Our brains are marvelous in creating new pathways, when we learn something new, we create new connections between our neurons.*

We are rewiring our brains to new experiences; this happens automatically however this is something that can also be stimulated. The ability to form new connections and change how the circuits are wired is called Neuroplasticity. There's also potential to replace the neurons that have died called Neurogenesis, which would be a whole new concept to revealing how we can prevent dementia or overcome brain injuries.

- *Learning a new language:* when we learn we are forming newer pathways in our brain, with each new lesson we can change the default mode of operation in our brain. Learning a new language or a musical instrument takes advantage of the amazing neuroplasticity of the brain. My journey to learning began when I happened to come across a post on social media that someone was offering to teach Spanish. I knew nothing about neuroplasticity or neurotransmitters or any of the background to learning and its connection to memory loss. I had an intuitive urge to seek out something that would create an excitement and make my brain active. I loved to learn or read about new ideas and concepts before I became unwell, but that spark had died down and I wanted to revive that. I was too fatigued to get ready and drive to my class but my love for learning kept me going. On the last day of my class my teacher happened to ask where I lived, she was amazed how far I had driven each week to learn. I did not even give it much consideration. So once you get yourself ready and out of the house it doesn't matter, you will always do what you need to do to make it work with this illness. The benefits of being bilingual really outweigh the other concerns we often have. Research shows that people who learned another language in adulthood exhibit less emotional bias and a more rational approach when confronting problems in their second language than in their native one. The heightened workout a bilingual brain receives can also delay the onset of diseases like Alzheimer's and Dementia by as much as five years. The bilingual brain also strengthened the dorsolateral prefrontal cortex, the part of the brain that plays a crucial role in executive function, problem solving, switching between tasks and increasing focus. When you take the first step to saying hello in a new language – Hola (Spanish), Bonjour (French), Guten Tag (German), Konnichiwa (Japanese), Namaste (Hindi) or more, you are saying hello to newer pathways in your brain.

- *Creating artwork:* art can boost introspection, memory, attention and focus. Any random sketches, doodling for few minutes daily or coloring, will help with stress, anxiety and calm your nerves too. At times even using the non-dominant hand to draw or write can make a huge difference to those brain connections.

- *Dancing:* enhances the neural connectivity and reduces the risk of Alzheimer's. Any form of exercise or movement helps release endorphins which provide pleasure and a feeling of euphoria. Motion always changes your emotion. When you learn to coordinate you are actually exercising your left and right brain. Initially I found my sense of coordination was way off, but eventually I learnt to train my brain to move in sync better. I'm still learning to get all coordinated, with more practice the better it gets.

- *Reading and expanding your vocabulary:* activates the visual and auditory processes as well as memory processing. Reading can be hard during brain fogged days; however, a daily reading habit of 5 minutes and gradually increasing it will help. Pick a book or a subject that really interests you and excites you so it will make the reading habit more enjoyable. Rich vocabulary has been linked to reduced risk for cognitive decline.

- *Playing puzzles, Chess, Sudoku:* doing puzzles reinforces the connections between brain cells and is effective for short-term memory loss. Playing games also involves fine motor skills which would help with hand and eye coordination. I used to play with my kids puzzles and felt I was getting my life back together one piece at a time.

- **Do math in your head:** doing math without using a pen and paper and mentally doing the calculations in your head, will help keep your brain active. Back in India, as kids we were never allowed to use the calculator until high school, all calculations had to be done mentally or on the paper.

Constant learning happens either by books, by attending classes or by taking a good hard look at your own life. When you fill up your brain with learning you automatically cut down the negative thoughts.

> *It's challenging to eliminate negative thoughts however these can be replaced with learning since we are training our brains to look at possibilities.*

It's easier to replace thoughts instead of suppressing or denying their existence. Learning creates the yearning to overcome struggles. What have been your past patterns in life when faced with a crisis? Through reflective thinking you can gain valuable lessons from it. Looking back when I had to face a problem or crisis situation, I always got into problem-solving mode. Getting to solve the problem was like solving a challenge, which gave me the energy to come up with solutions and actions steps. The more you reflect you might be able to identify your patterns. When we get to focus on the possibilities, we are stretching our brains to think further and beyond and learn to move past current disintegration.

I love the Japanese wabi-sabi philosophy which is all about celebrating impermanence, imperfection and incompleteness. The Japanese popular art Kintsugi, revolves around the same concept and involves repairing broken ceramics with gold alloy. This came up when the Japanese craftsmen were in search of coming up with an aesthetic way to repair the broken ceramics. Kintsugi highlights the strength and beauty in imperfection. When a ceramic object breaks, the Kintsugi art involves using gold dust and resin (or lacquer) to reattach the broken pieces. The final masterpiece incorporates the unique cracks into its design and the gold lines further enhance the beauty of the piece while strengthening it. The art form brings out the profound meaning for brokenness and healing – by embracing our brokenness and imperfections we create wholeness, beauty and strength. The broken object paradoxically becomes more resilient and more beautiful than ever before.

Similarly, our brains can go through fragmentation; we can reinforce and get it all back together by sprinkling the golden dust - our positive thoughts!

What's your MOTTO?

CHECK-IN

1. Do you ever feel brain fatigued, your attention span has decreased, you find decision-making difficult, lack attention or interest? Any of these or all of these?

_____
_____
_____
_____

2. What is one thing you are currently doing to reduce risk of cognitive decline?

_____
_____
_____
_____

3. What is one thing you would like to do to improve or retain brain health? (learn a new language, doodle, color, dance, exercise, read, play puzzles, do sudoku, play chess, etc.)

_____
_____
_____
_____

SUMMARY

• Our brains are marvelous in creating new pathways; when we learn something new, we create new connections between our neurons.

• The ability to form new connections and change how the circuits are wired is called Neuroplasticity.

• The heightened workout a bilingual brain receives can also delay the onset of diseases like Alzheimer's and Dementia by as much as five years.

• Mental health is one of the most ignored aspects in Hashimoto's. Learn to identify the symptoms early on so you can take action right away.

• When you fill up your brain with learning you automatically cut down the negative thoughts.

CHAPTER FOURTEEN

THE DIGITAL SUNSET MOTTO

Disconnection enables connection. During the day our brains are stimulated to a great extent with various sights, sounds, work, learning and communications. When we sleep the brain works on integrating the day's information inputs, by working on storing some of the information in the long term memory and deleting some of the files. Lack of quality sleep means the brain files are not stored in proper order. During the day the cognitive or executive functions are impacted since there was no qualitative data processing that happened overnight. The brain needs to be prepped to sleep better and to work efficiently.

Darkness signals our brains to go to rest. Our brains have a suprachiasmatic nucleus which works like a clock signaling the different body functions and various hormones to rest and recover. These hormones are triggered when the body senses light and works on the wake up mode activities. Our body clock works best when we synchronize with nature by adopting to rise up with the sun and to go to rest at sunset. Our brains do not differentiate between the sunlight and light from various other sources. **Using devices right before bedtime confuses the brain due to the light emitted from those devices and is further stimulated by the visual stimulus it receives and the neural networks get turned on for the action mode.** Instead of prepping the brain for sleep we are setting it up for a wake up operation.

During my motherhood days when I used to wake up to pump, I used to be on my phone - 30 minutes for each feed and 4 times at night meant I used to spend 2 hours at night on the phone. It was hard to wake up at night and I needed some sort of motivation which the cell phone provided. I used to go over all the photos and videos of my kids that I would have taken during the day or be on social media. However, getting back to sleep got harder too. My sleep cycle was already disrupted by frequent wake ups; little did I realize the harm of using a cell phone to stay engaged with my activity at night. With Hashimoto's I realized I used to feel exhausted and tired after a lot of computer and cell phone usage. On the cell phone I used to be on social media and the constant scrolling would worsen my carpal tunnel syndrome too. It was a blessing in disguise as I eventually controlled the usage of both. I used to have an allocated time to check my emails or use social media. I also noticed whenever I felt boredom that was the time I had the urge to connect to social media. We are at times so uncomfortable with the lack of excitement that we tend to reach for some stimulation through social media.

> *According to research, in the U.S. adults are now spending almost an average of 6 hours per day on videos.*

The alarming amount of time spent per week is close to 42 hours, as good as a second full-time job for many. That includes the time spent watching videos in an app or on a smartphone or tablet, as well as watching videos over a TV connected device like a DVD player, game console or on computer.

> *The average time spent on social media is 2 hours and 22 minutes per day.*

Cell phones, Wi-Fi routers, computers, blue tooth devices and microwaves send out a stream of invisible energy waves called the Electromagnetic frequencies (EMFs) and there is a concerning risk of radiation emitted from these devices. According to the World Health Organization's International Agency for Research on Cancer (IARC), EMFs are "possibly carcinogenic to humans." The IARC states some studies show a possible link between EMFs and risk of cancers in people. According to some scientists, EMFs can affect your body's nervous system function and cause damage to cells. EMF radiation from electronics interacts with the human body on a cellular level. This is because the human body also has its own electromagnetic field. Our blood, nervous and lymphatic systems all use electromagnetic signals as a means of communication throughout our entire body, for all of its basic and complex functions. This is why radiation can cause cellular mutations and cancers. One study states that "chronic exposure to electromagnetic radiation, at levels found in the environment, may particularly affect the immune, nervous, cardiovascular and reproductive systems."

Other symptoms of exposure to digital devices for longer periods of time may include:

- sleep disturbances, including insomnia
- headache
- depression
- tiredness and fatigue
- lack of concentration
- changes in memory
- dizziness
- irritability
- loss of appetite and weight loss
- restlessness and anxiety
- nausea

- skin burning and tingling

- changes in an electroencephalogram (which measures electrical activity in the brain)

There is often a gap or a lag between the time a person was exposed to the dangerous levels of EMF and the manifestation of its symptoms. Electromagnetic radiation at extremely low frequencies (so-called ELF) also provokes a stress response within the cells in the body. This can lead to chronic stress issues and eventually autoimmune responses. A person may also develop increased inflammation within the body after being exposed.

STEPS FOR DIGITAL SUNSET AND BODY RESET

- Turn down the lights in the home for an hour before actual bedtime. This will help increase the production of melatonin within the body signaling the body to get into rest mode.

- Digital devices such as cell phones can be turned onto the sunset mode or night time mode. This would reduce the amount of bright blue light emitted from the screen.

- Meditation, reading, journaling or calming music before bed helps the mind to mentally calm down.

- Massaging hands and feet or back of the neck and below the base of the head can help relieve some tensions from the body before sleep.

- During sleep the cell phones can be turned onto airplane mode which will help avoid notifications; Wi-Fi routers can be turned off at night

It's best if you can keep the cell phones in another room while you sleep, if this cannot be achieved an airplane mode might help.

During the day choose to use the head phones or use the speaker mode on the cell phone to talk instead of directly placing the phone over your ears. Some house plants are also said to avoid the radiations and purify the environment. Walking barefoot on beach sand has tremendous grounding benefits. Our bodies build up positive electrons in the form of free radicals when in direct contact with the ground as it neutralizes these electrons. In Japan, the government introduced the concept of shinrin yoku or 'forest bathing,' where citizens get to walk along with nature. It is believed to provide therapeutic benefits and Japan now has 62 designated therapeutic woods, attracting about 5 million visitors annually.

Once you get comfortable with turning off your devices for a few hours in the evening, see how you can extend the time period and see how much longer you are able to accomplish a digital detox. It's like fasting without the devices. Initially it could sound alarming, however, the more you learn to stay away from devices the greater you will enjoy the true benefits of human connection and thereby enriching your relationships.

What's your MOTTO?

CHECK-IN

1. Do you use your phone or watch TV before bedtime?
   _____
   _____

2. Are you aware of the number of hours spent on TV, social media, watching videos or being on the phone?
   _____
   _____

3. Have your ever felt your energy levels drain, or experience headaches, sleep disturbances, or any other symptoms with extended TV or phone usage?
   _____
   _____

4. Do you reach out for your phone the first thing in the morning as soon as you wake up?
   _____
   _____

5. What can help to reduce the hours spent on gadgets? (switching to airplane mode, leaving phone in another room while you sleep, keeping track of your time spent, etc.)
   _____
   _____

SUMMARY

• The brain needs to be prepped to sleep better and to work efficiently.

• When we sleep the brain works on integrating the day's information inputs by working on storing some of the information in long term memory and deleting some of the files.

• Darkness signals our brains to go to rest.

• Using devices right before bedtime confuses the brain due to the light emitted from those devices and is further stimulated by the visual stimulus it receives and the neural networks get turned on for the action mode.

• According to research, in the U.S. adults are now spending almost an average of 6 hours per day on smart phones, videos, television.

• Cell phones, Wi-Fi routers, computers, blue tooth devices and microwaves send out a stream of invisible energy waves called the Electromagnetic frequencies (EMFs) and there is a concerning risk of radiation emitted from these devices.

• Long term exposure to devices could cause fatigue, headaches, dizziness, sleep disturbances, lack of concentration, changes in memory, chronic stress and eventually autoimmune response.

• Learn to turn off your devices for few hours in the evening and see how you can extend the time period and see how much longer you are able to accomplish a digital detox.

CHAPTER FIFTEEN

THE REASONING MOTTO

Have you ever decluttered your home big time, gave things away or tossed them in the trash? How did you feel? The feeling of lightness and liberation, clearing up space, sense of accomplishment, the satisfaction of donating, you physically let go of your past items and thoughts associated with it, the simplicity in dealing with minimal stuff and then all of a sudden a greater sense of clarity. In the mind MOTTOs section, we saw how the mind can be made calmer with meditations, made smarter with exercises and rest and now we get the see how to bring about clarity by decluttering the mind. Similar to physical decluttering which clears up the space in the environment, the mental declutter helps with clearing up the mental space thereby providing tremendous clarity on how to focus on the important things that truly matter.

For the few years in my life living with brain fog and fatigue, I noticed I was unable to have the mental clarity and the decision making faculties which developed the urge in me to procrastinate. I would think through things so much that it would make me so brain fatigued and eventually I would end up brushing it aside and go to sleep. What some expert's term as 'paralysis of analysis' after intense brain strain due to overthinking, we end up doing nothing. Any unfinished activities or unresolved emotions would lead up to congestion and clog up your thoughts and weigh you down. It's crucial that we find an outlet and have things resolved to further progress in our journey.

BECOMING SUPER INTENTIONAL

There are two main factors that are going to take your personal wellbeing journey to a whole new level – becoming super intentional and making the commitment to healthy habits. Intentionality comes when we take a good hard look at what lies in front of us. However, if you find it overwhelming to initiate this, begin with a physical declutter which helps with mental declutter eventually. The physical decluttering even has tremendous psychological and mental health benefits.

> *Decluttering physical spaces leads us to being intentional. When you are grouping, sorting and rearranging and minimizing, you are mentally prioritizing by being intentional.*

An intentional life in one aspect of your life can easily be imported to all other areas of your life.

BENEFITS OF DECLUTTERING

• Having a decluttered pantry could demonstrate that you can be intentional in your health choices, because you know exactly what is there and you don't end up stocking items that may not be required.

• Clutter can cause stress since you need to go through piles of stuff to identify what you really need and makes it more disorganized. Research has linked less clutter to less cortisol, the stress causing hormone. Messy work and home spaces can leave you feeling overwhelmed, anxious and helpless. Day in and day out, and at night our brains organize and store brain files in order, this is something that happens to all of us that we are not conscious about. Brains prefer order and organized visual stimulus, when the visual distractions are high, there's brain drain due to a higher strain to make sense of what it views. We lose our ability to focus, drain our cognitive resources and also experience greater memory loss as we are not sure where we kept our belongings. According to the researchers at Princeton University's Neuroscience Institute, clutter makes it difficult to focus on one task or object. A disorganized environment drains your energy and defocuses your attention in different directions. When you declutter physically and mentally, since the brain is not forced to remember a lot of the unfinished business, you tend to sleep better too.

- Decluttering can make you happier and boost your mood and self-esteem. When you have an organized space you have a sense of accomplishment and a feeling that you have your life together.

- Decluttering brings a sense of gratitude when you notice the abundance of things you have in your life and also when you give it away it can make you feel altruistic. You might experience the physical benefits of space and the mental benefits of feeling more expansive.

- It can help with your financial troubles as well, as you know what you have, you are less likely to duplicate purchasing those items. Selling your items can bring in some extra cash and also you end up not having to pay for storage. In America the storage industry makes about $37.5 billion annually which means an average of $90 per month for the 1 out of 10 who choose to use it.

You will notice an increase in productivity, boost in creativity and save you a lot of time and effort in the long run.

There are many benefits to decluttering which is the first big step to becoming intentional. For me personally I had no trouble with decluttering my home space or organizing, my decision fatigue was what I had to work on. The best way to simplify the decision-making process is to commit to building healthy habits.

▪ *It's said an average person makes 35,000 decisions every day.*

What to eat? What to wear? What to do? The ideal way to save brain power is to minimize the number of decisions made every single day. Many successful people adopt this strategy and even wear the same outfits every single day. Barack Obama wears only gray or blue suits. Mark Zuckerberg sports his gray t-shirt and Steve Jobs was famous for his black turtleneck, jeans and sneakers. Obama said in one of his interviews, "you need to focus your decision-making energy. You need to routinize yourself. You can't be going through the day distracted by trivia."

MAKING THE COMMITMENT TO BUILDING HEALTHY HABITS

Real growth and transformation happens only with commitment backed by action, action here implies the discipline. Discipline provides the positive behavioral reinforcement to our brains when the set of actions are carried out day in and day out repeatedly, these later become the bedrock to developing great character. What you have read so far would be meaningless if there was no decision and then a commitment being made. The Mind MOTTOs have clearly highlighted how powerful our minds are and it's up to us to make good use of this super power we are all gifted with. When I look back at my life, I never lacked willpower or the discipline. So what really differentiates staying stuck with illness or having the mindset to recover and heal completely? It has a lot to do with the decision making ability. Willpower can get fatigued if we tend to depend on it every single time and keep using it, stretching our limits. The strength of willpower fades every time more decisions are being made.

▪ *The bottom line is to make a sound decision and back it up*

> *by action so we are not relying on willpower to get us through the situation.*

For example, not reaching for a bag of chips is easier if the decision to not eat it is made in the first place, instead of giving the mind two choices of should I eat it or not, thereby forcing a decision to be made at my end. Every time I have to make this decision it would cause more fatigue. On a day when the mind has a lot of decisions to be made, we tend to brush aside the choices that would actually make life better. A hard stressful day at work can eventually make us turn down going to the gym in the evening.

STEPS TO OVERCOME THE DECISION MAKING FATIGUE

- **Plan the previous night what needs to be done the following day**: I make my to-do list the night before and make sure simple decisions like what clothes to wear, what to eat etc., are taken care of earlier so I do not waste my mental power on these trivial aspects. I make a weekly to-do list every Sunday morning for the entire week. Kids activities, doctor appointments, paying bills are all scheduled in my calendar so I can plan the other activities around it. I also add going to the gym as an appointment so I do not skip it. My daughter once asked me if there were 'makeup' classes at my gym, I thought that was brilliant idea. If ever I happened to miss going to the gym Monday to Thursday, then I made sure I did make up for it by going on Friday.

- **The hardest gets to be the first:** The more complex or higher the priority the tasks, are the ones that need to be completed first thing in the morning. We simply have greater focus, and more energy in the mornings, so achieving the hardest task would give a greater sense of accomplishment and boost your self-esteem to ease accomplishment the other tasks with ease. My to-do list has a list of non-negotiable activities that appear right on top every single day – Yoga, Meditation, Walking, Gym, Reading and Gratitude (see more in The Golden Hour MOTTO).

• **Make the commitment:** Decisions get made only once, it gets backed up by commitment and action. Too many choices and too many decisions can leave us paralyzed and make us procrastinate. The decision to lose 30 pounds is made only once. Every single day we do not ask if we need to lose 30 pounds, what follows is a game plan and action steps to accomplish that goal. If you hope to make the right decisions every single day, you will fall victim to procrastination. When I had to deal with a multitude of symptoms I took a good hard look at all of my symptoms from head to toe, and wrote down every single one of them. I asked myself what are my current concerns, how would I like to feel as my final outcome and what are my current gaps, where I need to take the action to make my final outcome happen. Women tend to talk more than men, because we gain clarity when we get it all out. It's like sifting through flour, when we dump all the flour and sift, the best ideas emerge through the filter. Since I'm more of a thinker than talker, I love to think on white paper.

▪ ***There's magic in white paper and a simple pen.***

I dump everything onto the paper and keep thinking over it until ideas and action items emerge. Then I focus my efforts on getting those action items completed.

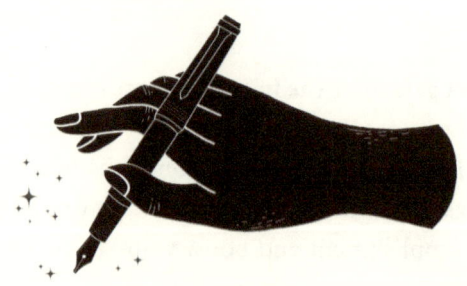

Below is how my chart looked, the gaps were the action items I needed to take to feel better. I focused on getting my action items done every single day and these were all scheduled in my calendar to make sure they were not missed out. Focusing on the process will eventually lead to the end goal.

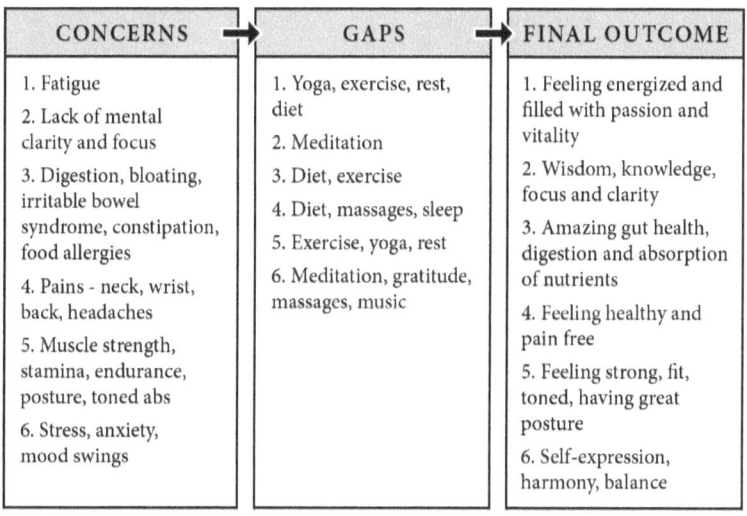

CONCERNS	GAPS	FINAL OUTCOME
1. Fatigue 2. Lack of mental clarity and focus 3. Digestion, bloating, irritable bowel syndrome, constipation, food allergies 4. Pains - neck, wrist, back, headaches 5. Muscle strength, stamina, endurance, posture, toned abs 6. Stress, anxiety, mood swings	1. Yoga, exercise, rest, diet 2. Meditation 3. Diet, exercise 4. Diet, massages, sleep 5. Exercise, yoga, rest 6. Meditation, gratitude, massages, music	1. Feeling energized and filled with passion and vitality 2. Wisdom, knowledge, focus and clarity 3. Amazing gut health, digestion and absorption of nutrients 4. Feeling healthy and pain free 5. Feeling strong, fit, toned, having great posture 6. Self-expression, harmony, balance

I once read that "the power of stories and the stories that we tell ourselves have the ability to keep us stuck. When we are able to reframe our inner stories, we are able to change what becomes feasible and what we can project ourselves towards and what we can actually accomplish. We are so busy thinking about the time we have and the possibility we don't have, but we need to think about the possibility we have and the time we don't. One day when we draw our last breath, the person we are gets to meet the person we could have become, our job in that blink of time, is to close the gap."

What's your MOTTO?

CHECK-IN

1. Do you feel the need to declutter or organize any aspect of your life?

_____

_____

2. Which areas of your life would you like to begin to organize or get more intentional about? (Health, Home, Relationships, Job, Finances)?

_____

_____

3. Do you have someone who can support you in the 'becoming intentional' process?

_____

_____

4. Write out your commitment statement to initiate the process.

    a. I _____ (your name) make the commitment today ____/____/____ (date) to get intentional about my _____ (your area of life that you want to change).

    b. Below are the top 3 action items I will do, starting today ____/____/____ (date)

    i. _____

    ii. _____

    iii. _____

5. My Reasoning MOTTO:

   a. My list of current concerns are (prioritize them):

   i. _____

   ii. _____

   iii. _____

   b. My final outcome (how you would like to feel):

   _____

   _____

   c. What are my current gaps (this is where you need to take the action to make my final outcome happen)?

   _____

   _____

SUMMARY

There are two main factors that are going to take your personal wellbeing journey to a whole new level – becoming super intentional and making the commitment to healthy habits.

• Physical decluttering clears up the space in the environment, the mental decluttering helps with clearing up the mental space, thereby providing tremendous clarity on how to focus on the important things that truly matter.

• Clutter can cause stress since you need to go through piles of stuff to identify what you really need and it makes it more disorganized. Research has linked less clutter to less cortisol - the stress causing hormone.

• It's said an average person makes 35,000 decisions every day. What to eat? What to wear? What to do? The ideal way to save brain power is to minimize the number of decisions made every single day.

• Decisions get made only once, it gets backed up by commitment and action. Too many choices and too many decisions can leave us paralyzed and make us procrastinate.

• What are your current concerns, how would you like to feel in your final outcome and what are your current gaps where you need to take the action to make your final outcome happen?

THE SOUL MOTTO

There would have been a stage in all of our lives where we might have gone through the search, wondering what next or where are we headed in our lives. It happens every time we are about to embark on a new chapter in our lives.

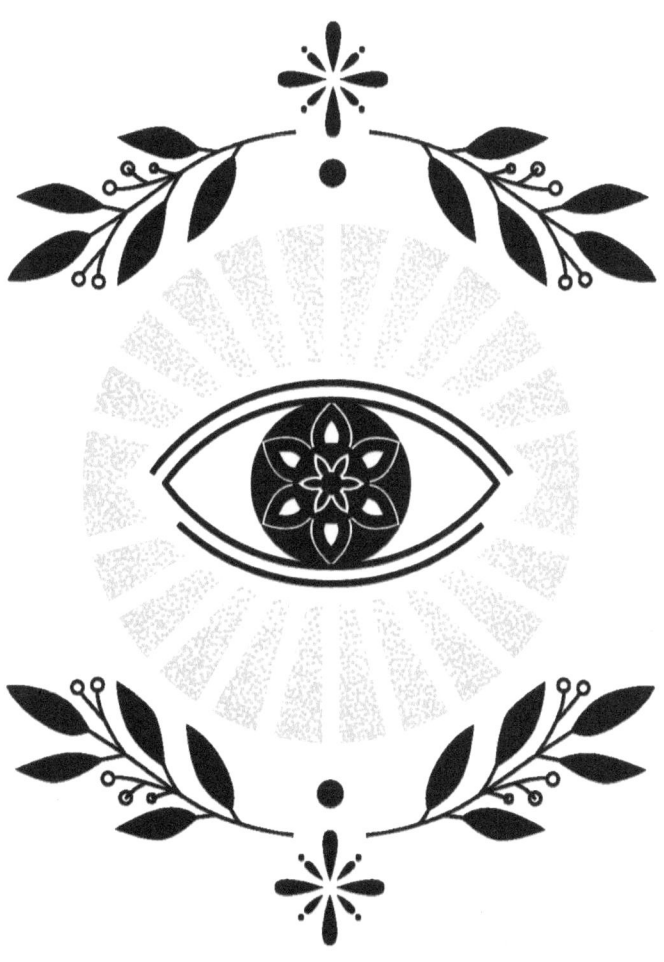

When we begin to think this is it, we are closer to knowing what we really want, there seems to be something new that comes up and shakes our belief of what we know. At each phase of life when we begin to realize that we have understood what life really means, the life phase changes. When the phase of life changes we realize that the meaning of life has changed as well. We begin to go around in circles with no real explanation and the perpetual search to understand continues. When we realize that the external searches yielded to nothing and the search is perpetual, that's when a new hope sparks within. We learn to connect within to know the answers and that is the true search that has just begun.

> *The deeper the well we dig within, the sweeter the water of knowledge we can receive.*

Soul MOTTO will help connect the dots and show the first steps in getting to know you in The Golden Hour MOTTO and The Supreme MOTTO.

CHAPTER SIXTEEN

THE GOLDEN HOUR MOTTO

The saying, "the longest part of the journey is from the head to the heart" is so simple yet so profound. As I was used to thinking a lot, getting to the heart seemed complex. I could even 'think' on this statement for a long time and wonder what might be the shortest route to the heart. Maybe if the head could travel a bit and the heart could travel a bit and they meet midway? Luckily, I did not have to think much then as I was too brain fogged to think anymore and it was also the time when I got into more of my meditation practice.

I loved the quiet time in the mornings with my coffee followed by yoga and meditation. I enjoyed it so much that I would look forward to it before I went to sleep the night before. I did not start off this way, what I got started on for 5-10 minutes every day gradually increased because I kept at it without skipping a day. I began to spend more time in yoga and meditation, I also began to read and listen to music which meant I needed much more time to finish up my morning routine before my family woke up, or else it would mean no quietness and me time. This drove me to wake up earlier than everyone in my family. There used to be a time when waking up early for me seemed an uphill task. I remember the day I got married, we had some early morning rituals to perform and I found it extremely difficult to wake up at 5 a.m. even on my own wedding day! I slowly began to wake up half an hour earlier and kept at it until I was able to make it to 5 a.m.

> *If there's a single MOTTO to pick for real transformation and growth it would be The Golden Hour MOTTO.*

There's phenomenal magic and vitality that the early morning hours provide. The more time we get to spend time in silence the more impactful it can be on our lives when practiced every day with dedication and commitment.

The brain produces several electrical patterns or waves. When we wake up at 4 a.m. the brain operates at 10.5 hertz per second. The range 8 to 13 hertz is called the Alpha stage - the gateway to subconscious mind. When you wake up early your mind is between alpha and theta stage and it is capable of deep and profound learning without you having to exert tremendous effort. Your mind is calm and not deep into thinking and you relax into the moment. The ancient yogis called this period the 'Brahma Muhurta.' Brahma means knowledge and Muhurta means time period, perfect to receive the knowledge which is an hour and a half before sunrise. The Brahma Muhurta is believed to add stability when yoga and meditation is practiced during this time. This is also the time when the pineal glands are at their peak, which means you can operate at your highest potential which helps with mental clarity, intuition, empathy, focus, optimism and decisiveness. For Buddhists the pineal is a symbol of spiritual awakening, in Hinduism pineal is the seat of intuition and clairvoyance, for Taoists it's the mind's eye and ancient Greek's described it as the 'sphincter of thought.' Many believe it's the seat of the soul where all thoughts are formed.

During the early morning hours your subconscious mind is highly impressionable and soaks up information like a sponge and whatever you see, hear or read will set the tone for the rest of your day. The brain can work at its maximum potential when it doesn't have to multitask. You can get to plan out your day and set goals without distractions and have the abundance of quality time during the day to work your plan. Successful people and high achievers take advantage of their brains function and capacity during these prime hours in the morning. The early morning wake routine discipline creates a whole day of discipline to achieve the goals. I feel more energized and more productive throughout the day when I get to finish my morning routine. Merely waking up early may not be the goal here, some get to wake up early with ease but they don't get to see significant impact in the quality of their lives. What we do during that time is what makes the difference and has the potential to change the trajectory of our journey.

THE GOLDEN HOUR ACTIVITIES

> *The Golden hour is meant to sow in good thoughts and positive mental attitude. What we sow in during the prime hours has tremendous impact on our attitude throughout our day.*

Deep seated thought patterns can be changed with a healthy early morning routine.

MUSIC

Music has tremendous power to help transcend you to another dimension. Studies show that music can create pleasurable emotions that light up the mesolimbic pathway, the reward part of our brain that cause those happy feelings. It's a great kick starter in the morning creating positive vibrations. The quietude can amplify the experience to greater extent. Listening to soulful music can make your day. Many religions have music as a way of offering their praise to the higher power. Music can calm the mind, energize you, enhance mental alertness, attention and memory and can even help manage your emotional and physical pains more effectively. You may choose any meditative music or instrumental songs to start your day. As you progress along your transformational journey you will begin to notice your musical preferences shift too and you get to enjoy more of calming classical music. As soon as I wake up and brush, I fix myself some coffee and sit down to listen to music and continue to listen to it throughout all of my activities during the Golden Hour.

READING

Reading can stimulate your mind and generate new ideas. Soaking in and absorbing all of the positivity when the mind is alert, can help you to stay positive during the day. One research revealed that reading can be like mental gymnastics for the brain. Reading influences our thought processes and is a very potent form of brain training. Reading is a great way to keep your brain fertile and is the best way to clear the negativity weeds. Reading anytime during the day helps, if you are not into reading early during the day, then you may choose to read some positive quotes and reflect on those thoughts which can take less than 5 minutes and can still have the same impact on your mood.

BRAIN DUMP

When the mind is full of thoughts, its best to empty it so you can fill it up with goodness. I feel like I'm mentally closing all of the browser tabs on my computer, one by one, and clearing up the memory space when I release it all out onto paper. Journaling for few minutes during the day is said to have therapeutic benefits. Writing during the early hours can reveal your inner desires, problems and even help with solutions. The Journal acronym according to the Coach Federation stands for:

J - *Judgement free* (safe space to express your thoughts and feelings)

O - *Observation* (you can step into an observer role by analyzing what you have penned down)

U - *Understanding* (what you observe can help you understand more about yourself)

R - *Revelation* (understanding about yourself can lead to revelations about your dreams, goals and aspirations)

N - *Needs Assessment* (writing daily can reveal areas that require assessment and help release your pent up emotions and feelings)

A - *Awareness* (the problem areas can be addressed with the first step of awareness)

L - *Life* (writing is an effective way to look at your life and learn from it).

YOGA, MEDITATION AND EFT

Once the mind is prepped with positivity through music and reading, thoughts that trouble us are emptied by journaling and so sinking into meditation gets easier and richer. Pranayamas or breath work can activate your prana or the life force. Ancient texts have stressed on the importance of early morning mind and body activation for enhanced longevity and wellness. Emotional Freedom Technique (EFT) tapping, also known as the psychological acupressure is believed to create balance in your energy system. Tapping on the key meridian points or energy hot spots in your body with your fingertips, helps relieve the disruption of energy, enhances mood and reduces depression. This can take only a few minutes and can be done prior to yoga or a meditation session and the results can be felt within days, and for some within minutes.

GRATITUDE, AFFIRMATIONS, VISUALIZATION

Gratitude helps acknowledge the goodness in your life and creates a mental shift by refocusing your thoughts on what you have instead of what you lack. Gratitude can improve your mood, provides a deep sense of satisfaction and even improves the quality of your sleep. Post meditation I find it an enriching experience to write out my gratitude. Writing down your gratitude and affirmations along with visualization after deep meditation, will make it flow easily for you. When I initially began this exercise, I told myself to pick three things I'm grateful for and I struggled to find those three things! I would write I'm grateful for the delicious coffee, a beautiful start to the day and an amazing potty experience (when you're down with Hashimoto's this can be a big thing to ask for!) for several months. I kept at it every day even though I felt I gained nothing from this exercise. After few months, I began to write more things I was grateful for. The list grew bigger and reached a stage where I began to write a full page of gratitude, affirmations and goals every day. As a person who struggled to find a few things to begin with, this exercise made me focus on and become more aware of the good in my life.

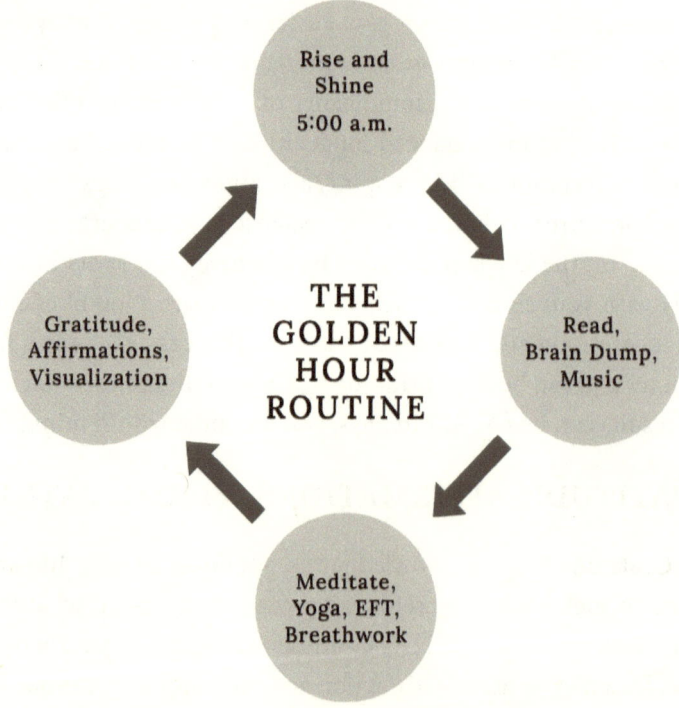

MY DAILY GRATITUDE LIST

Today I'm feeling grateful and wonderfully blessed, my heart is filled and overflowing with an abundance of _____

(love, peace, joy, happiness, stillness, ecstasy, bliss, oneness, spacious, expansive, meditative, spiritual, creative, self-expression, courage, knowledge, power, wisdom, truth, light, balance, harmony, guidance, intuitiveness, pampered, loved, secured, grace, glory, divine, kindness, compassion, poise, strength...)

I'm attracting amazing positive people, events, resources, opportunities that are in line with my true highest purpose.

I'm growing every day in every single way and becoming the best version of who I'm meant to become.

I'm leaving a rich legacy _____

(success, prosperity, courage, kindness, amazing human being...)

My purpose in life _____

(mine is helping people lead an intentional life)

My goals in life _____

Today's an amazing _____
_____ day!

(productive, purposeful, intentional, fun, love filled, joy filled...)

You may choose to begin with one of the above activities to start your day. Start for a few minutes and gradually increase as per your pace. Notice how you begin to feel by incorporating these in your daily routine.

Make a routine of waking up early and going to bed early. Between 10 p.m. to 2 a.m. is when you get the most regenerative and deep sleep. Sleeping later than 2 a.m. denies your body of the regenerative effects making you groggier during the day. You need to slow down physically and mentally before 10 p.m. so your body can get to utilize the melatonin. At 10 p.m. your body fully utilizes the effects of melatonin generated providing you with the much needed rejuvenation. If you typically go to bed after 10 p.m. start making those small shifts by getting to bed earlier by 15 minutes, then 30 minutes. Making sure you get to bed by 10 p.m. will help the body to wake up earlier. Before going to sleep I spend a few minutes with breath work, EFT tapping and massaging my feet and palms while listening to music. These are like book ends to the day, a great start and a good finish has greatly improved my quality of sleep and also sleeping as soon as I hit my bed.

Sometimes I used to go to bed later than 10p.m. on weekends and would wake up later, only to realize that I would feel wearier than usual. Waking up later would also disrupt my quiet time in the mornings as my kids would wake up and I would end up going through my morning routine faster so I could fix breakfast for them. The idea of having a nice sleep in on weekend mornings never worked at my household as my kids wake up earlier than usual on weekends than on weekdays. If I ended up skipping the morning routine, I could see the slump in my energy levels and also by midday, I would realize that I had hardly accomplished anything on my to-do list. The extra sleep in the mornings and the late nights were hardly worth the effort.

Choose consciously your tone of the day. A strong and consistent routine can help you find your purpose in life. Quietness connects us to our heart enabling us to hear the heart's whispers. One day these quiet whispers will be loud and clear if we continue to connect with silence. To find the quietness and stillness in this busy and fast paced world we need to carve out me time. When we are always on the move and doing, being in stillness feels uneasy and an uphill task initially. However, with gentle reminders and practice, we can get to the state of being and also follow nature's way of guiding us to the destination of stillness with a sunrise and sunset routine. By accessing stillness, we can then tap into the heart's desires and inner wisdom and be guided by it, which would bring about the balance in our lives. The mind can then help conceptualize, visualize and create strategies to manifest the desires of the heart.

What's your MOTTO?

CHECK-IN

1. What does your current morning routine look like?
_____
_____
_____

2. How would you like to change your routine? Which of these can you incorporate into your mornings? (Music, Reading, Brain Dump, Meditate, Yoga, Gratitude, EFT, Affirmations or Visualization? Choose any one to begin with)
_____
_____
_____

3. Can you adopt an early bed routine?
_____
_____
_____

4. What is the number one thing that can help you to get started with a healthy morning routine?
_____
_____
_____

SUMMARY

- If there's a single MOTTO to pick for real transformation and growth it would be The Golden Hour MOTTO.

- When you wake up at 4 a.m. your mind is in the Alpha stage which is the gateway to the subconscious mind.

- The early morning is also the time when the pineal glands are at their peak which means you can operate at your highest potential, which helps with mental clarity, intuition, empathy, focus, optimism and decisiveness.

- What you do after you wake up early is what makes the difference and has the potential to change the trajectory of your journey.

- What we sow in during the prime hours has tremendous impact on our attitude throughout our day. Deep seated thought patterns can be changed with a healthy early morning routine.

- Music can help you to transcend to another dimension. Music can calm the mind, energize you, enhance mental alertness, attention and memory and can even help manage your emotional and physical pains more effectively.

- Reading can be like mental gymnastics for the brain. Reading influences our thought processes and is a very potent form of brain training.

- Brain dump and journaling for few minutes during the day is said to have therapeutic benefits. Writing during the early hours can reveal your inner desires, problems and even help with solutions.

- Pranayamas or breath work can activate your prana or the life force.

Ancient texts have stressed on the importance of early morning mind and body activation for enhanced longevity and wellness.

• Emotional Freedom Technique (EFT) tapping, is also known as the psychological acupressure and is believed to create balance in your energy system.

• Gratitude helps acknowledge the goodness in your life and creates a mental shift by refocusing your thoughts on what you have instead of what you lack.

• Quietness connects us to our heart enabling us to hear the heart's whispers. One day these quiet whispers will be loud and clear if we continue to connect with silence.

CHAPTER SEVENTEEN
THE SUPREME MOTTO

Awareness initiates the wonderful process of deep inner connection. When we begin to connect the various elements of mind, body and soul, we develop better understanding on the greater purpose in life. Life's unexpected changes can leave us stifled in uncertainty, insecure and puzzled on what really matters and what we need to focus on. The first step to this great journey begins from awareness. Connection then becomes the bridge, helping you to cross over with a leap of hope and courage, leaving the life's challenges beneath.

The more we understand inner connection the greater will be the realization on how we can learn to connect better with minds, people, hearts and everything. You are going to tap into the innate wisdom and indomitable inner strength which will open the doors to new beginnings in life. **Hashimoto after all, means base of the bridge. 'Hashi' means bridge and 'moto' means base. This illness could mean the bridge or the connection to an awakened life.** Each moment could be strengthening your inner bridge to the Supreme power. Maybe this bridge could stretch and take you across many miles, teaching many valuable life lessons. You can choose how you respond to what happens to you, you are not at the mercy of what has happened. When you choose to look beyond and know you can recover, this is the first step of awareness. This awareness can lead you to respond and take control. You regain your power and resilience when you choose to take control and you are not giving your power away to external circumstances.

Pain is the fuel to succeed and achieve greatness. The greater the pain, the greater will be the determination. It's part of the larger plan so that one can achieve greatness. Look back on anyone's journey and when was the time the greatest growth happened? It was in moments of intense resistance to move forward. When did you marvel and feel good about yourself? Even the smallest step forward then, needed the greatest courage. Change can be hard, but will determine it's possible, irrespective of however stuck you might feel in the moment. Resilience may not even mean going against the current, it could be choosing to slow down and deepening that inner connection to thrive. The greater the hurt, the greater the creative out lash - be it writing, poetry, artistry or music. It's the key that unlocks your soul's greatness. Creativity is expressing oneself. Spirituality is experiencing oneself and beyond. When you experience, you need to express, and you express more effectively only through your experience. What began as lack of self-expression in the form of this illness, ultimately transformed me and gave me the courage to express myself. Connecting the dots as to what could be a better purpose than this? Every illness and pain has a much larger purpose that takes time for us to comprehend and in the end it leads us through a process of self-discovery and transformation if we choose that path. When I felt I lacked 'the energy,' it took me through a journey across several miles. It taught me the transformational power of stillness and brought me back to my source and the realization that energy cannot be destroyed, it can only be transformed. I was in search of managing my fatigue and energy and looking for several outside factors, but it broke down my thought patterns, altered my thinking, and gave me the realization that my indomitable energy was well within myself and I had to tap into it.

When life forced me to slow down, I'm grateful I chose self-love.

The intense self-love created the shift within me, I was on a quest to learn more and understand more of the purpose. I felt restless and deeply unsettled that there was more to life and I could not figure out the purpose. I used to wake up early, listen to music, do my yoga, and then get deep into meditation and once done, I used to write and make sketches, write down every single thing that came into my mind right after my meditation. Some of the questions that popped up in my mind then were:

a. What do I love to do?

b. What frustrated me?

c. What did I want to change?

d. Who do I love to be with?

e. Who are the leaders I greatly admired?

f. Why did I admire those people?

g. What qualities in them did I admire?

Some of these questions were the beginning to understand myself better. These could be the clues to identifying your soul's purpose as well. Or it might lead to several other questions that might mean something to you. Every day the meaningless scribbles continued, I would read and listen from morning until night. I knew something was missing and did not know what exactly it was. Movies, television, and social life - nothing interested me. As I limited my exposure to the outer world, my inner world blossomed. I was searching for answers during my meditations until one day I had a thought to write a book. When I came out of my meditation, I broke into a sweat since it felt like a lofty goal and I had never written before, I had no idea what to write about and strongly felt this was not something for me. I brushed it aside thinking it could be some random thought that came to me during my meditation. I continued to search and was restless, months went by, and it seemed like a mirage; every time I felt I was getting closer to realizing the truth, the further it went. The thought to write a book occurred a few more times and after one session I felt that I had to achieve this. The more I ignored the thought of not writing, the more agony I felt. I made the decision, sat down and looked at a blank piece of white paper. My mind was blank as well, I wrote down a few questions; if I need to write who should I get in touch with and what could I write about? I did not have any of the answers on the how-to's, however, my why was strengthening and deepening with the sessions. The courage to think on the lines of writing was strengthening. Connecting to the stillness can make you courageous to take the risk and get yourself out of the comfort zone big time. Once the mental clutter slowly dissipates with meditation it reveals the real you. Sometimes the revelations show us a newer 'you' can be possible and the mind takes time to accept the new reality.

How can we know what really is the purpose then? When something really comes from deep within and pours out from your heart and soul. Just thinking about it will make you want to cry, do something, take the action, it creates the sense of urgency and gives you the tremendous power to accomplish it no matter what the circumstances are. It wrings your heart and tugs your soul. Sometimes it could just be a flicker of a dream but when you continue to work on it, it builds momentum and gathers tremendous energy needed to manifest it. In the beginning when you start off, it could just be you, for you, but it expands in a great way that it then becomes all encompassing. Working towards helping others and making sure they don't get to endure the same pain as you did. The only thing on your mind will then be the cause; to make sure that no else has to endure that. Everyone has a calling and you evolve as a person through your purpose.

> *How would you know your calling? You wouldn't and the world wouldn't know unless you take the chosen path.*

You were given certain talents, certain circumstances to help you choose your calling. To accomplish your purpose, you need to have the push and the pull. When you are pushed and pulled into all directions, you cannot realize your heart's real push and pull. Becoming the person you were meant to be, requires dusting the soul and taking a good look at your heart's desires. Keep your motivations in front of you, they will lure you but you may not progress much. Keep the motivations within you and they will move you to your destination effortlessly. When the motivations lie deep within then you begin to eat right, exercise right and all of the other body and the mind MOTTOs fall in place, one by one, since these are not the external drivers and these have now become the non-negotiables in your journey to reach the Supreme soul MOTTO. Caring and self-love becomes the bedrock to your success as you need the mind and body functioning at its best to help the soul reach its purpose.

I once read that the unexamined life is not worth living, but also know that the unlived life is not worth examining. **You were not meant to be a spectator - you are here to be spectacular. The real wellbeing comes when the soul magnificently awakens.**

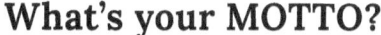

What's your MOTTO?

SUMMARY

- Awareness initiates the wonderful process of deep inner connection.

- Hashimoto after all, means base of the bridge. 'Hashi' means bridge and 'moto' means base. This illness could mean the bridge or the connection to an awakened life.

- You can choose how you respond to what happens to you. You are not at the mercy of what has happened.

- Pain is the fuel to succeed and achieve greatness. The greater the pain, the greater will be the determination. It's part of the larger plan so that one can achieve greatness.

- The intense self-love created the shift within me, I was on a quest to learn more and understand more on the purpose.

- Connecting to the stillness can make you courageous to take the risk and get yourself out of the comfort zone big time.

- Everyone has a calling. You evolve as a person through your purpose.

- Becoming the person you were meant to be, requires dusting the soul and taking a good look at your heart's desires.

- You were not meant to be a spectator, you are here to be spectacular.

AUTHOR'S NOTE

Dear MOTTO-ers,

We started the journey together as Hashimoto-ers and we now end on a transformed new MOTTO-ers, as you take charge and define the way you love to feel and be. I hope this book is the self-help guide to help propel you through your journey forward. While writing this book, every day my thoughts were to make sure that I did not miss out mentioning anything that really helped me to recover. I had to overcome the severe memory loss issues to make sure I did not miss out anything. Reminiscing the period in my life where I struggled did not come easy, as I could not recollect the moments. What kept me going was my burning desire to help you and give you the belief that you too can recover.

If you are in the process of recovering, I would love to hear from you and how you are doing at the moment and how this book is helping you. What are your areas of struggle, where do you need help?

If you have recovered and become stronger and reached the other end, I would love to hear from you. What were the MOTTO's that you adopted? Is there anything else that you did outside of the MOTTO's listed that you would love to share with the community?

What's your MOTTO?
www.meenachan.com

ACKNOWLEDGEMENTS

I'm grateful and thankful to my adorable kids Kavin and Tara who mean the world to me, they are my energizers, my fuel to succeed and my constant source of inspiration to becoming who I'm meant to be.

I'm thankful to my husband Aravind, who has been a pillar of support all throughout and who always believed in me.

My parents and my in laws who have been great role models to me, providing unconditional love and warmth.

I'm ever so grateful to Samantha Houghton my coach, mentor and editor for her love, patience, support and for bringing out the best in me with her constant words of encouragement.

To Meher Rajpal who brought life to my book with her beautiful artistic expressions. What cannot be captured in words has been brought out beautifully through her illustrations.

NOTES

Chapter Two

    1. When Depression starts in the neck, Harvard Health Publishing, July 2011

    2. American Thyroid Association on postpartum thyroiditis

    3. Hopkins medicine on postpartum thyroiditis

    4. Piedmont Healthcare on hyper and hypo thyroid

Chapter Three

    1. American Thyroid Association on postpartum thyroiditis

    2. Cleveland clinic medical professional, Hashimotos, June, 2020

Chapter Five

    1. TCM Body Clock: why do we wake up or feel ill certain time of the day? Organic Olivia, 30 OCTOBER, 2014

Chapter Eight

    1. What happens to your body when you walk 10000 steps, Mary Bowerman, USA TODAY Network, Apr 15,2017

    2. Why walking is the most underrated form of exercise, Brianna Steinhilber, NBC news, May 4, 2018

Chapter Nine

    1. Do you yoga: doyou.com

Chapter Ten

    1. Leaky gut: what is it, what does it mean for you? Marcelo Campos, MD, Harvard Health Publishing, September 22, 2017

Chapter Eleven

1. Ayurverdic texts on what is marma therapy

2. Drmariza.com on essential oils

Chapter Thirteen

1. The truth about Hashimoto's and Brain Fog, Dr. Joni Labbe

2. The benefits of a bilingual brain by Mia Nacamulli

Chapter Fourteen

1. Should you be worried about EMF exposure? Erica Cirino, Healthline, March 7, 2019

Chapter Sixteen

1. This is why billionaires wake up at 4 a.m. by Be Inspired.

2. 5 Transformative methods to activate your pineal gland and tap into your superhuman potential, Scott Jeffery

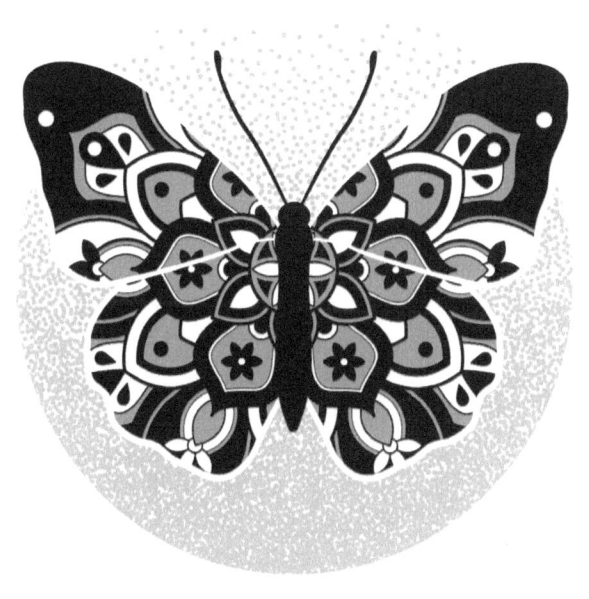

www.ingramcontent.com/pod-product-compliance
Lightning Source LLC
Chambersburg PA
CBHW031109080526
44587CB00011B/900